RISING TO THE CHALLENGE OF LIFE AFTER CANCER

Rising to the Challenge of Life After Cancer: Expert Advice for Finding Wellness is an easy-to-read self-help guide for people facing cancer diagnosis and treatment. Following an effective Q&A format and based on a unique Wellbeing Essentials framework, it offers a valuable 'dip in and out' approach with signposting to evidence-based guidance on major challenges that those diagnosed with cancer and their family and friends may face. If you or someone close to you has had a cancer diagnosis, then this book is for you.

With a focus on wellness and taking control, questions addressed include 'Is there a best way to cope with cancer?', 'What strategies can help me make an informed decision about treatment?', 'What is prehabilitation and how can this help me?', and 'Who am I now?'. The book covers an array of essential guidance from maintaining social health and wellbeing to accessing care and support in the community. It is written for both those living with or beyond cancer as well as their support network. The book also includes Jeff and Suzanne's personal stories about their lived experience of cancer and a Resources and Connections section with tips for further information and support.

Written by academic experts who are also 'experts by experience', this book is indispensable for people with cancer and their families, and anyone wanting to understand more about the condition, as well as health and social care professionals and students of social care, health care, and nursing.

Jeffrey Charles Dunn, AO (Officer of the Order of Australia), is Professor of Social and Behavioural Science and Chair of Cancer Survivorship in the Division of Research and Innovation at the University of Southern Queensland, where he leads research into strategies to improve survivorship outcomes for people affected by cancer. Alongside this, he is Chief of Mission and Head of Research at the Prostate Cancer Foundation of Australia. Jeff's focus is the connection between research and practice, working closely with leading academics and clinicians across the country to change policy and practice to improve outcomes for people affected by cancer. Jeff is the Immediate Past President of the International Union for Cancer Control based in Geneva. Jeff was appointed an Officer in the General Division of the Order of Australia in 2014 for distinguished service to medical administration through leadership roles with cancer control organisations and promotion of innovative and integrated cancer care programmes.

In August 2022, Jeff was diagnosed with a stage three rare and aggressive Blastoid Mantle Cell Lymphoma, for which he received an autologous stem cell transplant and has ongoing therapy.

Suzanne Kathleen Chambers, AO (Officer of the Order of Australia), is Executive Dean of the Faculty of Health Sciences at the Australian Catholic University. She is a registered nurse and practising health psychologist who has worked as a practitioner and researcher in psychological support for people with cancer for over 30 years. Professor Chambers is an Officer of the Order of Australia for distinguished service to medical research, particularly in the area of psycho-oncology, and to community health through patient care strategies for people with cancer.

Jeff and Suzanne are life partners and, in this book, they connect their professional and personal experience to provide pragmatic and evidence-based advice about common challenges after a cancer diagnosis.

'The strength of this book – aimed at helping people with cancer, their families and loved ones – is the authenticity that comes from two cancer professionals who have been through, and are still going through, dealing with cancer themselves either as patient or partner, reaching out to share their objective knowledge along with their personal experience.

These authors set the standard for how to write about coping with cancer by bringing together the weight of their many years of professional experience with their personal journey. A very helpful book to guide others through the emotional, social and physical maze that cancer presents. I highly recommend it.'

Adjunct Professor Maggie Watson PhD. DipClinPsych. AFBPS.
Editor Emeritus: Psycho-oncology: Journal of Psychological, Social and Behavioral Dimensions of Cancer and Associate Fellow British Psychological Society

'Despite all the advances in cancer diagnosis and treatment, or perhaps because of them, navigating a myriad of challenges after a cancer diagnosis, can be an overwhelming task for the person with cancer and their family. The stakes could not be higher. And while the technical information on treatment types and side effects is increasingly available, the more existential questions of what this illness means to me, my life and my loved ones, often remain unanswered.

Enter *Rising to the Challenge of Life After Cancer: Expert Advice for Finding Wellness* – a concise Q&A style guide to some of these questions, written by a pair of experts in supportive care in cancer who are also experts through lived experience of facing the cancer diagnosis themselves. The guide explores key issues of meaning, normality, identity, relationships, and flourishing with honesty, courage and a touch of self-deprecating wit, that is so uniquely Australian. This is not a sanitized scholarly manuscript – this is the story that touches deeply at emotions. As a result, the words of advice are not only convincing because of their grounding in evidence, but also because of their authenticity.

It takes courage to take a great personal challenge, like a cancer diagnosis, and use it for a greater good. Professors Dunn and Chambers have done just that, and we are all better for it.'

Professor Bogda Koczwara AM BM BS FRACP MBioethics FAICD she/her.
Senior Staff Specialist, Department of Medical Oncology, Flinders Medical Centre. Professor, Flinders Health and Medical Research Institute, Flinders University

BPS ASK THE EXPERTS IN PSYCHOLOGY SERIES
BRITISH PSYCHOLOGICAL SOCIETY

Routledge, in partnership with the British Psychological Society (BPS), is pleased to present BPS Ask the Experts, a new popular science series that addresses key issues and answers the burning questions. Drawing on the expertise of established psychologists, every book in the series provides authoritative and straightforward guidance on pressing topics that matter to real people in their everyday lives.

All books in the BPS Ask the Experts series are written for the reader with no prior knowledge or experience. For answers to everything you ever wanted to know about issues important to you, ask the expert!

Managing Your Gaming and Social Media Habits
From Science to Solutions
Catherine Knibbs

How to Live Well with Dementia
Expert Help for People Living with Dementia and their Family, Friends, and Care Partners
Anthea Innes, Megan E O'Connell, Carmel Geoghegan, and Phyllis Fehr

Understanding and Helping to Overcome Exam Anxiety
What Is It, Why Is It Important and Where Does It Come From?
David W. Putwain

Rising to the Challenge of Life After Cancer
Expert Advice for Finding Wellness
Jeffrey Charles Dunn and Suzanne Kathleen Chambers

For more information about this series, please visit: BPS Ask The Experts in Psychology Series – Book Series – Routledge & CRC Press https://www.routledge.com/our-products/book-series/BPSATE

RISING TO THE CHALLENGE OF LIFE AFTER CANCER

Expert Advice for Finding Wellness

JEFFREY CHARLES DUNN, AO (OFFICER OF THE ORDER OF AUSTRALIA), AND SUZANNE KATHLEEN CHAMBERS, AO (OFFICER OF THE ORDER OF AUSTRALIA)

Routledge
Taylor & Francis Group

LONDON AND NEW YORK

First published 2025
by Routledge
4 Park Square, Milton Park, Abingdon, Oxon OX14 4RN

and by Routledge
605 Third Avenue, New York, NY 10158

Routledge is an imprint of the Taylor & Francis Group, an informa business

British Library Cataloguing-in-Publication Data
A catalogue record for this book is available from the British Library

ISBN: 978-1-032-63882-9 (hbk)
ISBN: 978-1-032-63881-2 (pbk)
ISBN: 978-1-032-63884-3 (ebk)

DOI: 10.4324/9781032638843

Typeset in Joanna
by Apex CoVantage, LLC

Access the Support Material: www.routledge.com/9781032638829

CONTENTS

FOREWORD

In May 2022, I was in Geneva attending a board meeting with Jeff Charles Dunn, the President of UICC. As we walked back and forth between the hotel and the office, I noticed that Jeff, usually so full of enthusiasm and energy, wasn't quite himself. Then (a few months later), in mid-August, Jeff shared the difficult news – he had been diagnosed with cancer.

Cancer is a journey no one ever anticipates, but for those who face it, it changes everything. Through my work with the Swedish Cancer Society and UICC, I've met countless individuals and families affected by this disease. Each story is different, but they all share one common thread – the profound impact cancer has on both the person diagnosed and their loved ones.

Every year, 20 million people receive a cancer diagnosis, and the number continues to rise. Some of this increase can be attributed to positive factors – people are living longer, giving more time for cancer to develop, and advances in detection mean we are better equipped to find cancer early, improving the chances of survival. However, an increasing number of cancer cases are also linked to lifestyle choices, adding another layer of complexity to cancer control.

Over the years, I have read many books by those who have faced cancer, each offering a unique perspective. However, this book stands apart. Written by Jeff Charles Dunn and Suzanne Kathleen Chambers, both respected researchers and individuals who have personally faced cancer together, it blends scientific insight with deeply personal reflections in a way that few others do.

This book is more than just a guide – it is a companion. From the moment of diagnosis through treatment and beyond, it provides clear, practical advice for navigating the complex and often overwhelming landscape of cancer. But, what truly sets it apart is the honesty and vulnerability with which Jeff and Suzanne share their experiences. The reflections at the end of each chapter are raw and heartfelt, serving as a powerful reminder that cancer doesn't just affect the body; it touches the heart, mind, and soul.

At times, the book also captures the almost absurd, comical aspects of daily life amidst a cancer diagnosis – like when one of them runs a simple errand only to receive a life-changing phone call from a healthcare provider, forcing an immediate, important decision. A cancer journey is filled with thousands of such small, unexpected moments, and it's easy to feel lost along the way. But in the company of Jeff and Suzanne, you won't feel lost.

Their story is a testament to resilience, love, and the importance of support and understanding. Whether you are a patient, a caregiver, or someone close to someone with cancer, this book will guide you, encourage you, and remind you that you are not alone on this journey.

Jeff and Suzanne have poured their knowledge, experiences, and hearts into these pages. I believe their words will touch many lives, offering comfort, insight, and hope to those who need it most.

With deep respect and admiration,
Ulrika Årehed Kågström
President of UICC, Union of International Cancer Control (and
Secretary General of Cancerfonden, the Swedish Cancer Society)
Stockholm, October 2024

ACKNOWLEDGMENTS

This book distils 30 years of work into insights we hope you will find valuable in nurturing wellness after a diagnosis of cancer.

It would take another book to name all of the people we wish to thank, including the many friends and colleagues who reached out to us after Jeff's diagnosis. You know who you are – we have maintained our own wellness in large part thanks to your support.

In the writing and editing process, the assistance of colleagues Samantha Clutton, Anne Savage, Nicole Heneka, Rob Newton, and Daniel Galvao was invaluable. So, too, was the energy and enthusiasm of our teams at the University of Southern Queensland, Australian Catholic University, Prostate Cancer Foundation of Australia, and the Union for International Cancer Control.

To our four children and two grandchildren, who remind us every day that wellness is a way of being – we are grateful to be in your embrace.

And thank you, our dear reader, for kindling the hope that inspires us to continue caring.

THE AUTHORS

WHO ARE WE, AND WHY ARE WE GIVING YOU THIS ADVICE?

The treatment of a disease may be entirely impersonal; the care of a patient must be completely personal. One of the essential qualities of the clinician is interest in humanity, for the secret of the care of the patient is in **caring for the patient**.

Francis W. Peabody M.D.
– Journal of the American Medical Association (1927)

We have dedicated our careers to caring for the patient and encouraging policy makers, practitioners, and researchers to do the same – to consider the patient and not just the disease. As partners in life and partners in the quest to improve outcomes for people with cancer, we stand as a force. As our horizon of knowledge expands, the quest for quality of life rises to stand alongside the preservation of life itself. Each of us, in different but connected ways, has pursued the goal of ensuring health and medical science bring measurable benefits to the lives of individuals, their families, and communities. At the core of what we do is the philosophy of person and family centred and driven care, directly connected to best practice and an evidence base.

Jeff's story:

I am currently Professor of Social and Behavioural Science and Chair of Cancer Survivorship in the Division of Research and Innovation at the University of Southern Queensland, where I lead research into ways to improve survivorship outcomes for people affected by cancer. Alongside this, I am Chief of Mission and Head of Research at the Prostate Cancer Foundation of Australia. In this role, I lead prostate cancer survivorship research but also play a connecting role between research and practice, working closely with leading academics and clinicians across the country to change policy and practice to improve outcomes for men with prostate cancer.

Over the course of my career, I have published more than 170 peer-reviewed manuscripts and numerous chapters and reports; received more than $37 million in grant funding; been an invited speaker at innumerable national and international conferences; and led and chaired various international meetings and workshops. I am in the top 2% of scientists worldwide for oncology and clinical medicine (Ioannidis, John P.A. 2024; DOI:10.17632/btchx-ktzyw.7). I have led research translation in psychosocial care in oncology through distress screening and stepped care models on a state, national and international level. I have developed and steered numerous partnerships between universities and community-based non-government cancer control organisations seeking to harness the power of both for changes that will improve outcomes for cancer patients and their families. I am a past Director, Board Member, and Secretary for the International Psycho-Oncology Society and an Editorial Board member of Psycho-Oncology Journal of the Psychological, Social and Behavioral Dimensions of Cancer. Following my interest in peer support as a method of care delivery, I am Scientific Adviser and Past Chair of the Reach to Recovery International Breast Cancer Support Service.

In 2019, I co-edited with Suzanne a special issue, "Re-Imagining Psycho-Oncology", in the European Journal of Cancer Care with a focus on stimulating innovation in psycho-oncology, including new technologies, methodologies, novel targets, and theoretical approaches. In 2022, I co-edited a special issue, "Global Psycho-Oncology", in the *Psycho-Oncology Journal of the Psychological, Social and Behavioral Dimensions of Cancer* with a focus on research emanating from lower-and-middle-income countries.

More recently, I led the development of a framework for cancer survivorship that includes as the central domain personal agency, explicitly placing the patient and their family at the centre of care. The other five domains are Health Promotion and Advocacy, Shared Management between the patient and the health professional, Evidence-based survivorship interventions, Care Coordination, and Vigilance. Taken as a whole, these domains propose an approach to guide the provision of integrated quality cancer survivorship care across all care settings.

Initially, my work in cancer began in community-based cancer control, where I led the development of programmes in health promotion and cancer survivorship with a focus on accessibility. This included initiating programmes to deliver accessible cancer information and support to people affected by cancer through a statewide Cancer Helpline, as well as psychological support through a Cancer Counselling Service that delivered clinical psychological care services both face-to-face and through telehealth or remote delivery. In this work, I co-authored the first published stepped or tiered model of psychological care for people coping with cancer. A tiered model of care articulates between need, distress, and depth of care. As needs increase, the depth of care increases and the intervention focus narrows and becomes more specialised. The goal is to ensure people get the right support at the right time, matching care to need.

I have led the development nationally and internationally of structured peer support programmes for people with cancer, recognising the value and importance of shared experience as a buffer to stress and a coping resource. Parallel to this, I pursued community-driven advocacy on cancer control, resulting in changes such as legislative control of solaria and passive smoking protections, doubling of government support to assist people from rural areas travel to major centres for their treatment, and policy change to provide cancer researchers access to population-based cancer data. My interest in reducing disparities in cancer outcomes for people who are socio-economically disadvantaged or for whom geography exists as a barrier to cancer treatment and care has been a driving force in my work in Australia and internationally.

Globally, I have worked as a volunteer for the Union of Internationally Cancer Control (UICC), based in Geneva, for more than 20 years. The Union for International Cancer Control represents the world's major cancer societies, ministries of health, patient groups, and influential policy makers, researchers, and experts in cancer prevention and control, with a membership base of over 1,200 organisations in 172 countries. The organisation leads and convenes capacity building and advocacy initiatives that unite and support the cancer community to reduce the global cancer burden, promote greater equity, and ensure cancer control continues to be a priority in the world health and development agenda.

My involvement in the UICC since 2002 has included leading as Chair of the Asia Pacific Cancer Society Training grant programme (2002 to 2016) and taking sustained leadership roles as a member of the World Health Organisation Non-Communicable Diseases Task Force, the World Cancer Leaders' Summit steering group, the City Cancer Challenge task force, and as a mentor for the SPARC programme (Metastatic Breast Cancer) project grant. From 2022 to 2024, I took on the globally elected role of President of the UICC to lead the major international cancer control efforts of this organisation, working with health and medical research groups across the globe, including the WHO International Agency for Research on Cancer, Cancer Research UK, City Cancer Challenge, McCabe Centre for the Law and Cancer, Asian Pacific Organisation for Cancer Prevention, Lancet Commission, to name a few.

As President of the Union for International Cancer Control, I spearheaded international collaborations towards the implementation of health and medical strategies that promote realisation of the United Nations Sustainable Development Goals and foster harmony and wellbeing worldwide. Over the past three years, this has included major initiatives designed to safeguard the health of the world's First Nations peoples and steer the global pandemic response in the area of cancer control. This includes my high-level leadership of a coalition working to improve Access To Oncology Medicines (ATOM) and personal involvement in recent initiatives delivered by the World Health Organisation to amplify the lived experience of people with cancer and the impact of antimicrobial resistance on cancer control.

At the national level in Australia, I was Appointed an Officer in the General Division of the Order of Australia (AO) 2014 for distinguished service to medical administration through leadership roles with cancer control organisations, and to the promotion of innovative and integrated cancer care programmes. This award is related to my work in developing major initiatives in cancer research as well as the development of policy and infrastructure to support cancer control.

Suzanne's story:

I started my career as a Registered Nurse working in intensive and coronary care. I moved to community-based cancer control three decades ago and found my passion in working with people affected by cancer. Following this passion, I graduated as a psychologist in 1995, and in 2004, completed a doctoral degree in psychology. I specialise in psycho-oncology as a researcher and practitioner. My work in the community included developing and delivering psychoeducation programmes for people with cancer, supporting peer support programmes in breast cancer, brain tumour, and prostate cancer, and supervising the delivery of psychological care interventions to literally thousands of people with cancer and their carers.

My research and practice in this area included remote delivery of care through telephone and internet-based programmes and support for couples where one partner was diagnosed with cancer. In my work, I have utilised a range of cognitive behavioural approaches, including acceptance strategies, mindfulness-based cognitive therapy, problem-solving therapy, and decision support. My work in the community continued until 2011 when I moved to the University sector, first as a researcher at Griffith University, then Director of the Menzies Health Research Institute of Queensland, to Dean of Health at the

University of Technology Sydney and now a national role as Executive Dean of Health Sciences at the Australian Catholic University.

I have won numerous awards, including being an Australian Research Council Professorial Future Fellow, William Rudder Fellow, and leading a National Health and Medical Research Council Centre for Research Excellence in Prostate Cancer Survivorship. I have published more than 300 peer-reviewed manuscripts, many reports and book chapters, and four books.

I am an Officer of the Order of Australia for distinguished service to medical research, particularly in the area of psycho-oncology, and to community health through patient care strategies for people with cancer. Along with Jeff, I am in the top 2% of scientists worldwide for oncology and clinical medicine (Ioannidis, John P.A. 2024; DOI:10.17632/btchxktzyw.7).

In 2021, I took on the role of Executive Dean for the Faculty of Health Sciences at the Australian Catholic University (ACU). This national Faculty includes three Schools: Nursing, Midwifery, and Paramedicine; Allied Health; Behavioural and Health Sciences, and is one of the largest Health Faculties in Australia. The mission of ACU, acting in Truth and Love, a commitment to human dignity, and the pursuit of knowledge reflects my aspirations in research and health care practice and is one I am dedicated to. The Catholic intellectual tradition of pursuing knowledge through both faith and reason resonates well with the challenges of facing a life-threatening disease and the perspective shift that this often involves.

I am a Fellow of the Australian Psychological Society College of Health Psychologists, and I currently practice as a health psychologist specialising in cancer and chronic disease.

Underpinning my approach as a psychologist is the centrality of a trusting, non-judgemental, and compassionate relationship between the therapist and the client, where the client feels safe to explore their challenges, grow to understand their strengths and pursue new ways of being if they so wish. My aim is to assist people to maximise their wellbeing and move towards valued personal goals by integrating elements of acceptance, commitment, and self-compassion into the therapeutic conversation.

I regularly present in national and international webinars on cancer survivorship and have written self-management books for men with prostate cancer and their partners that have been widely endorsed by health care professionals and consumers nationally and internationally. I have co-written with Jeff guidelines for health professionals on delivering psychological care for people affected by cancer. I am frequently called on to train health professionals in this area of care and have done this on a national and international level.

Our story:

We have both worked in cancer control for more than three decades, sometimes together and sometimes apart. Our shared commitment to this work over the years has provided the opportunity to partner with many dedicated health professionals and community groups in different ways.

In 2018, we established an Australian-based not-for-profit group, Open Eyes Global, as an incorporated association to support children with cancer in Nepal. To achieve this, we partnered with Nepal civil societies, directing funds to the Tilganga Institute of Ophthalmology in Kathmandu to provide customised prosthetic eyes to Nepalese children who have had their eye or eyes removed to treat retinoblastoma. Without this support, these children suffer lifelong facial deformities and stigmatisation. In 2022, Open Eyes Nepal was established in Kathmandu to partner with Open Eyes Global and formally take on local leadership in advancing care for these children. This work is an ongoing passion and commitment for us both.

In 2022, Jeff was diagnosed with a Stage three aggressive and rare blastoid mantle cell lymphoma. Given eight weeks to live without treatment, he underwent several months of intensive chemotherapy followed by a stem cell transplant. He is now in remission and having maintenance immunotherapy. With his wife Suzanne at his side, he continues his work in cancer control and has shared his own cancer diagnosis in the print and electronic media and internationally at the

World Health Organisation and the UICC World Cancer Congress to promote the advances in treatment driven by medical science while also strengthening the consumer's voice and highlighting issues of equity in cancer care nationally and internationally.

Between us, we have four daughters to whom we are devoted, each pursuing their own careers in education, journalism and global food security. We have two grandchildren, twin girls, who we adore. We breed Australian Lowline Cattle, a breed originally derived from Aberdeen Angus, and share a love of the natural world.

Professor Jeffrey Charles Dunn AO and
Professor Suzanne Kathleen Chambers AO

1

WHAT AM I FACING?

FACING CANCER

Experts from the International Agency for Research on Cancer estimated that across the world, 19.3 million people received a diagnosis of cancer in 2020. (1) These same global experts predict that by 2040, this number will have risen by 47% to 28.4 million new cancer cases. So somewhere in the world, every day, and every minute, a person will be told they have cancer. For most of us, we do not expect this to happen, and even as we undergo medical tests and procedures and the outcome seems clear, we hope for different news.

In mid-2022, our lives took an unexpected turn. Jeff was preparing to meet with Australia's Health Minister, lobbying for cancer research and survivorship care, and I was travelling internationally in my work as the Executive Dean of Health Sciences at a large Australian University. Jeff had developed a prominent swelling in his neck and, for the first time in his 40-year career, had to attend the meeting at the Federal Parliament without wearing a necktie. Shaking the Minister's hand self-consciously, he made light of the faux pas. Within weeks, he was diagnosed with Mantle Cell Lymphoma. It was rare, aggressive, advanced, and incurable.

Jeff soon began a treatment regime that continues today, starting with four rounds of intensive chemotherapy and an autologous stem cell transplant.

DOI: 10.4324/9781032638843-1

If you have experienced cancer, or if you are the companion of someone who has, then we have written this book for you.

It is about hurting, and hope.

WHY ME?

There is no answer to 'why me'. Some of us may have risk factors that increase our chance of being diagnosed with certain cancers; there are cancers that are associated with lifestyle factors, and others have genetic links, but for many cancers, no cause or connections are known. Cancer is, in many ways, a non-discriminating disease; it can happen to anyone. And if you or someone close to you has received a diagnosis of cancer, there is work to do.

We are fortunate that treatments for cancer have evolved and become more effective over time, and with new advances in medical research, treatments are continually improving, bringing new hope. As a result, people with cancer in many countries are now cured of their cancer, and if not cured, will live longer. Cure and increased longevity can come at a price, though, and treatment side effects can be mild or, in other cases, bothersome, long-term, and life-changing. Cancer is now often described as a chronic disease, which is a very different perception and perspective from how cancer has been viewed historically.

How you perceive your cancer diagnosis, and what it means for your life and who you are, will to a large extent be an unfolding narrative as you move through treatment and rehabilitation. The purpose of this book is to raise questions that might be important for you to think about now and into the future, to discuss what is known about how to help yourself have your best possible outcome, and ultimately to find your focus and turn your energies towards what matters to you most.

At the outset though, as you read this book and you work through the challenges ahead, we suggest that a morsel (or two) of self-compassion is helpful. You don't have to 'get over it' or become a 'better person'. Looking after yourself and your needs is a better option. Finding and activating your personal strengths and support networks and being informed will be important. As will being an advocate for yourself or your loved one.

IS THERE A BEST WAY TO COPE WITH CANCER?

A diagnosis of cancer is a major life stress. Finding out that you or your loved one has cancer is for most people a shocking experience. Cancer is a threat to survival, to a person's sense of self, lifestyle, and future hopes and plans. All seems at risk when facing a cancer diagnosis. Anxiety, feelings of shock, anger, loneliness, sadness, and depression are not uncommon reactions.

One way of understanding our responses is to think of cancer and the medical experiences that go with it as a threatening situation or event. When we experience a threatening event, our bodies react in a way that is designed to help us fight or flee. Put simply, if we are in a situation of threat, our sympathetic nervous system activates a hormonal response that triggers in our body a very rapid, generalised, and systemic response. This is an automatic physiological reaction that from an evolutionary point of view is designed to help us survive dangerous situations. When this response is triggered a range of physiological changes occur with the goal of getting your body primed to run or to fight. Your heart and respiration rates go up, pupils dilate, certain blood vessels constrict, and others dilate; it is quite a list. If you are told you or your loved one has cancer or that you need major and potentially life-threatening medical treatments, then this reaction is very likely. Except that there is no one to fight, and it won't help to flee, so you are left with unpleasant bodily sensations that we generally will label as anxiety, fear, or even panic.

This is important to know so that if you find yourself experiencing these types of physical or somatic reactions, you might take it as a sign to yourself to stop for a moment and consider what is happening in your life right now. From this, you can start to plan how you might best look after your own wellbeing.

So, is there one best way to cope with a cancer diagnosis? The central point to remember here is that individuals differ and will have their own preferred ways of coping with challenging situations. Being judgemental towards yourself about how you are coping simply adds to the burden. At times, the situation you are in will call for a problem-solving approach, where clearly identifying the problem, strategies to solve the problem, and garnering the resources and support you need to do this is the best way to go. At other times, an emotion-focussed approach that aims to relieve feelings of distress and generate feelings of pleasure and joy will be more appropriate. The approach that is less helpful generally is avoidance. Avoiding issues might help you feel better for a short period of time, but in the longer run, it can be a block to solving problems and garnering support. And paradoxically, the problem you are avoiding will often become even more aversive as you run from it. We talk about this more in Chapter 4.

WHAT DO I NEED TO KNOW ABOUT MY CANCER?

We all have different preferences for how much information we need or want about the cancer diagnosis and how involved we want to be in making decisions about treatment. The time of finding out about the cancer is usually when anxiety is at its highest, so this can be the time when it is hardest to take it all in. Over time, your preferences for information and involvement in decisions may change, as well as your level of confidence in asking questions and advocating for yourself.

Cancer is not one single disease, and even within one general type of cancer, there will be different types. Understanding what type of cancer you or your loved one has, how aggressive the cancer is, and how advanced it might be helps you to understand what treatment options are possible. It also helps to get clarity on what information is relevant to your personal situation. Friends and family can sometimes offer advice to you based on their own previous experiences with cancer that actually have no relevance to what is happening to you. Being informed can help put well-meaning but unhelpful advice into perspective.

When it comes to treatment options and making decisions, some people like to be very involved, while others may prefer to take their lead from their treating oncologist or surgeon. In Chapter 2, we discuss decision making strategies that may be useful in working out your preferences and how to enact these.

Knowledge about treatments and the side effects that may occur helps you to make informed treatment choices, to prepare, and give yourself the best chance of managing any side effects while supporting the effectiveness of your treatment plan. Pre-habilitation (or *prehab*) is a term used often in sports science to describe exercises and steps taken by athletes to help prevent sporting injuries. In cancer, pre-hab means doing preventative health behaviours to reduce side effects, contribute to quicker healing, and even enhance treatment effectiveness. Being informed about pre-hab for your particular cancer treatment is important, and research shows it makes a difference in recovery. One way to think about it is to give yourself your best sporting chance towards your best possible outcome.

Pre-habilitation guidance will be specific to the type of cancer you have and the treatment you receive, so expert advice on side effects and evidence-based strategies to combat these are needed. Examples of pre-hab include pelvic floor exercises to support urinary or bowel continence, prescribed resistance exercises to build muscle mass, dietary and exercise programmes to lose or gain weight, and cognitive behavioural strategies to manage stress and build resilience. Health professionals who can give advice here include all members of your treatment team, including specialist nurses, allied health professionals such as physiotherapists, exercise physiologists, dietitians, and psychologists.

WHEN CAN I CALL MYSELF A SURVIVOR?

The most widely accepted definition internationally of a cancer survivor is any person who has been diagnosed with cancer. This term emerged back in the 1980s in North America from a community of people who had experienced cancer themselves and wanted to advocate for more holistic cancer care beyond medical and surgical treatments. The term survivorship refers to the experience of having cancer, and the idea of 'survivorship care' is for a person's care to include all aspects of their quality of life after diagnosis. So the idea is that cancer survivorship care commences from the point of diagnosis and extends for the whole of life and is centred on the needs of the person with cancer and those close to them. This is called person-centred care. Person-centred care can be hard to achieve. Health care is often provided around the needs of the health system and the processes that work for a treatment centre, rather than what works best for the individual. This is why understanding and knowing what you or your loved one needs and advocating for yourself is important.

You may not feel like the term cancer survivor works for you, and there is no reason you need to think about yourself in this way. Put simply, this term resonates for some people and not for others. What is important is to approach your care in a way that pays attention to what matters for you and what will help you achieve your best possible health state. And whether you call this a survivorship plan, or a well being plan, is beside the point.

JEFF'S REFLECTION

Evidence suggests that most men and women, though we may suffer health anxieties, underestimate the likelihood that we will be diagnosed with cancer. I was no different and was not expecting to be diagnosed with Mantle Cell Lymphoma at the young age of 64.

We are narrative beings, and my diagnosis was not part of the narrative I had ever imagined for myself. Suzanne was in the garden when she learned the news, and I was in the hardware store, distracting myself from what I feared was coming.

In the days and weeks afterwards, I was inundated with messages of support and heartfelt expressions of solidarity from around the world – an outpouring of concern from friends and acquaintances gathered over a lifetime of work in cancer control.

And yet, I felt alone, suspicious of myself for this weakness, this capitulation to disease, while fearful of an uncertain future for me, my wife Suzanne, our family, and a career that had given definition to my life and work.

After decades of researching the psychological impacts of cancer, my own diagnosis hit home with a deeply disconcerting truth: cancer had stripped me of agency. I was not prepared and could not have been, and I found myself at the mercy of the medical system.

Theoretically, I know what agency is – a sense of control – essential to effective care, but the question of how to restore it had never seemed so perplexing.

More so for the fact that I am male, concerned with matters of providing, being, doing – averse to sympathy, wary of pity, and avoidant of every nuance of neediness that cancer imposes.

And I know I am not alone. Over many years, I have spoken to countless men diagnosed with cancer who, not knowing where to turn, retreat inwards, self-isolate, resist.

In this context, and notwithstanding good intentions, the question 'How are you?' can be confronting. We want to be fine, but we are not, and so we obfuscate, we fumble with words, and we pretend.

We are, after all, only human. But if cancer has taught me anything, it is that we are stronger than we realise. I am here today as proof of that fact and offer you that hope.

SUZANNE'S REFLECTION

I was watering my vegetable garden when the haematologist called me to tell me of Jeff's diagnosis. Jeff had just received his call with this news while he was at the hardware store, so we were each on our own. This wasn't ideal. But the situation was serious, and urgent decisions needed to be made and fast action taken. To say the least, I was shocked, devastated, very distressed, and my immediate reaction was one of rejection of the news. I just simply found it hard to take it all in, and my response to the advice that a stem cell transplant was needed was to push back immediately. I knew what that treatment entailed, I understood the physical toll it would take on Jeff, and I wasn't having any of it.

I must say Jeff's doctor was pretty patient and accepting of my strong response (strong words were used), and by the end of the conversation, I had moved on to accepting what needed to happen and to planning how best I could support Jeff and how we could get through this together. This became my complete focus.

It was only a few days before Jeff was admitted to hospital to start treatment. From my perspective, this was all very anxiety producing and challenging. And I now as a health psychologist who works with people facing cancer had to take my own advice. I still have moments where it all seems surreal to me, and when I suddenly find it hard to breathe (very strong fight-flight response). I try to look at my anxiety with interest and see what it has to teach me. And you have to hold tight to hope. Not always easy.

Being informed about what you can do to help yourself and your loved one is crucial. This gives you options to consider, a plan of attack, a course to follow, and a re-consideration of future goals and what matters most. Flexibility matters, and not sweating the small stuff as much as you can. And hang on tight.

REFERENCE

1.   Bray F, Laversanne M, Sung H, et al. Global cancer statistics 2022: GLOBOCAN estimates of incidence and mortality worldwide for 36 cancers in 185 countries. *CA Cancer J Clin.* 2024; 74(3): 229–263. doi:10.3322/caac.21834.

2

IS THERE A BEST WAY TO MAKE DECISIONS ABOUT MY TREATMENT?

MAKING DECISIONS ABOUT TREATMENT

It wasn't until the late 1980s and early 1990s that the idea that patients should be involved in decisions about their cancer treatment started to gain traction. (1)

Before this, people diagnosed with cancer often had limited involvement in the decisions about their cancer treatment. A passive decision making role where the surgeon, physician, or oncologist plotted the course ahead and put the plan into action was common, and the layperson adhered to the plan (or at least tried or appeared to). In cancer, the change to more patient involvement in their treatment decisions also coincided with the emergence of consumer-based cancer advocacy, most notably in North America with the formation of the National Coalition for Cancer Survivorship in 1986. (2)

Currently, shared decision making is seen as the ideal way for a person to make a decision about their medical care. The idea of shared decision making is that the patient is involved in their treatment decision to the extent that they desire, are supported in making the decision by their treatment team and people close to them, they are informed about their options and the consequences of these different options, and finally that they are enabled to make a decision

DOI: 10.4324/9781032638843-2

guided by their own personal values. The goal is for the patient to make a decision that supports their personal autonomy and that is arrived at by a process of mutual consensus with the clinician. This is a worthy goal, but it can be hard to achieve. Some decisions about treatment are straightforward and seem obvious. However, when there are multiple treatment options of equal or similar effectiveness or when the side effects of treatment are significant, making a decision can be challenging.

WHAT MAKES DECISION MAKING ABOUT CANCER TREATMENTS DIFFICULT?

There are a number of reasons why making decisions about cancer treatment can be stressful and confusing.

First up, the point of diagnosis is generally when a person's levels of distress and anxiety about their cancer are greatest. They will be trying to understand the implications of their cancer and what it means for their life now and for their future plans and hopes. When a person is anxious or distressed, it can be hard to think through decisions, and people tend to pay attention more to negative stimuli and imagine negative outcomes more than positive ones. (3)

They might also feel time pressured to make a decision. In some cases there may be urgency to start treatment to obtain the best possible outcome, and this increases feelings of pressure and stress. In other situations there will be time to reflect and consider different options; however, from this, feelings of uncertainty and discomfort seem prolonged. Many of us find uncertainty in itself an unpleasant state, and so being expected to take time to think things through, consider different options, and make a critical life decision becomes stressful in itself.

Adding to this, the medical jargon used by doctors is, for most people, unfamiliar. Terms like 'targeted immunotherapy', 'autologous stem cell transplantation', and 'radiation oncology' are not everyday language and while most of us know what chemotherapy is, the range of drug names used varies, even when it is actually the same drug.

Clinicians also sometimes use terms that are in and of themselves scary to hear. The proposal of 'lethal dose' chemotherapy followed by a 'rescue procedure' is hard to hear, as is hormonal ablation or chemical 'castration'.

Finally, there is always some level of uncertainty about the effects of the treatment, usually expressed as risk percentages, which in themselves can be difficult to interpret. Risk percentages are based on studies from often large groups of people with the same or a similar cancer. They tell you what has happened previously in studies of groups of people, but these statistics cannot tell you for sure what will happen to you as a unique individual. There will always be a range of outcomes that different people experience, even with the same cancer type and the same treatment, so some uncertainty always persists. As well, if the risk is presented as 'relative risk' this can seem misleading. For example, if you are told that having a certain treatment will halve or reduce your risk of cancer recurrence by 50%, that sounds impressive. However, if your actual risk of recurrence is only 10%, then reducing this by half to a 5% risk of recurrence sounds very different. So, relative risk needs to be balanced with information about the absolute or actual risk for you in order for you to be fully informed.

IS THERE A BEST WAY TO MAKE DECISIONS?

There are different theories about how people make decisions in real life. One approach is to categorise decision making as either heuristic or systematic. (4)

Heuristics are decision shortcuts or 'rules of thumb' that allow us to make a choice quickly and with minimal mental or cognitive effort. By contrast, systematic processing involves gathering information and weighing up the options to make a decision. It takes more effort and takes longer to do.

As an example, deciding on treatment based on a previous experience and the memory of that experience is called the 'availability heuristic'. This is a heuristic rule based on a readily recalled memory.

The problem with this approach can be that the memory that comes to mind may or may not be relevant to your situation. The expert opinion heuristic is where a person might rely entirely on the advice of their clinician without considering the options. It is not necessarily a bad strategy, but it may mean the person later on down the track wonders if they made the best decision for them and if they perhaps should have considered other options. Decision regret is always possible after any medical treatment, but strategies to avoid this through a deeper consideration can be helpful.

Systematic decision making involves seeking information and being informed about the options, weighing up the pros and cons of the different options, and, from this, making a decision based on personal values or priorities. This takes more time and more cognitive effort than using a 'rule of thumb'. So it is more effortful and time consuming at a time when you might feel like you just want to get on with treatment and move forward.

Many people will use a combination of systematic and heuristic processing to make their decisions. Either way, being informed will help you be better prepared for treatment and take steps to prepare and self-manage any treatment side effects. So, knowing what is ahead matters.

WHAT STRATEGIES CAN HELP ME MAKE AN INFORMED DECISION ABOUT TREATMENT?

The first step is to be clear about what decision you need to make right now. One thing you can be sure of is that there will be more than one to make either now or over time. So, getting clear about this and prioritising the decisions you need to make and addressing them in turn can help with not getting quite so overwhelmed. As you do this, ask your doctor for guidance on how quickly they think you need to make these decisions and build this into your decision making strategy.

Once you are clear about the decision or decisions you need to make, the order in which you need to make these decisions, and the time frame, think about who can support you in your decision.

Having a trusted person with whom you can talk over what is happening can help you to process the content of what is going on and also reduce a sense of being alone. So think about enlisting the support of a close friend or family member. If possible and you are comfortable with doing so, have this person sit in on medical consultations. This provides an extra pair of ears to take it all in and to check your understanding in the days and weeks to come.

Some people also find it helpful to discuss the decision with someone who has had a similar cancer experience. There will always be differences between their situation and yours, but support from a peer with personal experience provides a different perspective from family and friends and from the health care team. You may have people in your own social networks who have had a similar experience, and many cancer organisations in the community offer peer support to people and groups you can connect with. Details of these are included at the end of this book in a section called *Resources and Connections*.

Alongside this, think about how involved you want to be in the decision and let your clinician know how much information you need and what your main concerns are. Your health care team cannot read your mind, so your guidance on this is important to help them meet your needs. It is also useful to let the team know who your decision support person is and who you want included in the conversation about treatment.

WHAT DO I NEED TO KNOW ABOUT AND CONSIDER?

The next step is to work out what information you need to make the decision and then consider your choices. Your doctor and health care team should have provided you with some written information about this alongside their verbal explanation. Many countries have community-based cancer societies that also provide information. A good example is Cancer Research UK, which has a website, chat forum, and nurse Helpline that is freely available. Many other countries have similar services, and some are specific to certain cancer types. Once you have all the information you feel you need, you are well placed to consider your options.

A simple, workable approach is to list the treatments you are considering and write down the pros and cons of each approach. Once you have done this, draw a circle around the pros and cons that matter most to you personally. This may give you a sense of the direction in which you are leaning in your decision. It might also help crystallise what your main priorities are in making your treatment decision. Now think about the different pros and cons you have noted down, and consider if any of these can be influenced by steps you can take. For example, if there is a side effect you are most worried about, what can be done to prevent or ameliorate this? If there are practical considerations such as needing to travel for treatment or the extent of time off work, can these problems be eased by support from others or assistance from your workplace? Try using a problem-solving approach when thinking about each of your key concerns and seek information about these from a reliable source. Now review the pros and cons again, talk it over, if possible, with your support person, and then again circle what matters most to you. If you do this in an iterative process, your strongest preference should become clearer.

WHAT ELSE MIGHT HELP?

Other tips are to record what is said in consultations with your doctor either on your phone or by writing notes. If you do this, you can then check with the doctor that your understanding is correct. Often, you will find questions arising in your mind *after* you have seen the medical team – write these down so you can ask for clarification at your next appointment. When keeping notes it helps to have them in a book so you don't lose them and can refer back when you need to. People often say they get swamped with information, so start a file for all of this to help you keep track. If you feel unsure and would like a second medical opinion, then ask your doctor to arrange this. Think about what you feel you need in your health care team and work as hard as you can to organise this.

The system is not always your friend in this process. Health systems are organised around how they can efficiently process patients and get the work done. I think we all understand this as necessary, at least in part. But it also means that your specific needs might go unnoticed and unmet. Learning to be your own best friend and advocate is crucial here. Go hard or go home is an idiom about putting in the effort. We know you are exhausted, but in this situation, the effort is worth it.

JEFF'S REFLECTION

From the get-go, a cancer diagnosis brings baggage. Plenty of baggage, myriad things unexpected and unwanted yet nagging for attention and, for many, for a decision.

My earliest recollection of a decision was taking a call from my Haematologist on a Friday morning, the day after a battery of tests and biopsy, sporting bruised veins and a bandaged neck. I was in the local hardware store, distracting myself while waiting for results. So, I answered the phone:

"Hello Jeff, I have results. Are you able to talk?"

"I am in the hardware store."

"Would you like to talk now, or can I call back when you get home? What would you prefer?"

There it is. A decision. What would I prefer? How do I know what I would prefer? Kind of depends on what the news is, how long it will take to deliver, what the implications are, who I might need to contact immediately after or not, and the list goes on, including how many others are nearby in this public space and how I might react.

"Sure, let's do it."

I learned I had a rare, aggressive cancer that, even if treated successfully, has a habit of coming back, so the objective is to get into remission and then keep it there – all this while in the adhesive's aisle of the hardware store.

"We need to get started with treatment right away. I have arranged for you to be admitted to the hospital on Sunday. Is that okay?"

"Sure."

There it is, another decision.

And so it went . . .

Decision after decision, and they kept coming. Important each one and made on the fly in emotionally crowded and rationally compromised circumstances. Yet, with few exceptions, they needed to be made with little space or time for rumination.

I remember an organisational psychology class I took as an undergraduate student and a decision making model, FIDO, useful for practical deployment to improve outputs in business. I liked it; that is why I remembered it – simple with a straightforward, linear logic. Essentially, when looking to improve outcomes, remember that Feelings may negatively impact Information, which then may compromise the quality of Decisions, leading to poorer Outcomes. Therefore, dealing with feelings and emotions will lead to improved outcomes; conversely, not dealing with them will lead to poorer outcomes. The problem is with cancer: how do you easily deal with the feelings and emotions, the fear, the pain, the grief, the uncertainty? You can't, not really. You just can't. Well, I couldn't.

The message, individuals are different from organisations, and as individuals, we are all different from each other. There is no right or wrong way, no formula, no guarantees. We need to make the best decisions we can with what we have on the table in front of us in the circumstances we find ourselves. Canvass the health care team, trusted others, and those who love us, and do some research if time permits. Even so, it can be a messy, sloppy affair, textbook flawed. Nevertheless, decisions need to be made, and once made, outcomes need to be managed; that is the fact of the matter. Make the best decision you can under the circumstances and manage the outcome.

I would like to offer some inspirational quotes about decision making, which are countless if you Google them. Mostly they seem trite and unsuitable, to my mind, when it comes to a cancer diagnosis, with a focus on business or relationships, or self-actualisation, rather than survival, upside down Maslow. Though Nelson Mandella, through dint of his own hardship, offers consolation in what might usefully serve as a toast. So, to borrow from Mr Mandella, a toast to those diagnosed with cancer, "May your choices reflect your hopes, not your fears". That's my tip when it comes to decisions – if unsure, choose hope.

By the way, the best decision I made on that Friday morning on the phone in the hardware store was to tell my Haematologist to call my wife and tell her everything that he had just told me. She would have questions that I had not thought about, I would get details jumbled, and I just needed her to know before I got home, so it was best to call her. He did, and she swore quite a lot, I am told. But she did ask questions and sort the details, and together, we took it from there. That was a good decision.

SUZANNE'S REFLECTION

My job while Jeff was deciding about treatment was to support and keep him safe as much as I could. Having said that, not overstepping was important. These were his decisions to make, and the consequences would happen to him, not me. So I was really respectful of that and of the boundaries for him as a person and as a man.

I went to every clinical consultation, took notes in my bright red treatment book, and asked questions when I could tell by a nod of Jeff's head that it was my turn and it was okay for me to butt in. I started a file with all the paperwork we were given and read everything so I could sign post for Jeff if this was something he needed to be across or if he could leave it with me. I was very comfortable with stepping up and being assertive on his behalf when this was needed, but always with his agreement.

I did do a bit of background checking by looking up the research and reaching out to people we knew who I thought were knowledgeable and sensible. This was really to help me as a supporter rather than trying to influence the process. The more I knew, I figured, the better I could stand beside Jeff in all of this and back him up. We had a friend connection that led to a communication with someone who had a similar cancer experience to Jeff, and I was able to test this out to see if it might be helpful, and it was. In some ways, I was the semi-permeable barrier to the world where the priority was getting Jeff well.

Friends and family are your solid base and protective force in facing cancer, but moderation is sometimes needed. As a life partner, this was something I could do. I did have my days, let me tell you, when I was so exhausted and weighed down with trying to get it right. And hope seemed hard to really grasp. But what got me by were humour, Jeff and I working as a team, a few hidden tears, some great female friends, and our lovely daughters.

REFERENCES

1. Waldron T, Carr T, McMullen L, Westhorp G, Duncan V, Neufeld S-M, et al. Development of a program theory for shared decision-making: A realist synthesis. BMC Health Services Research. 2020;20(1):59.

2. National Coalition for Cancer Survivorship; 2024. Available from: https://canceradvocacy.org/.

3. Hartley CA, Phelps EA. Anxiety and decision-making. Biological Psychiatry. 2012;72(2):113–8.

4. Pravettoni G, Gorini A, Bonanni B, Veronesi U. The role of heuristics and biases in cancer-related decisions. Ecancermedicalscience. 2013;7:ed26.

3

WHAT IS PREHABILITATION, AND HOW CAN THIS HELP ME?

WHAT IS PREHABILITATION, AND HOW CAN THIS HELP ME?

Prehabilitation is a term that is often used to describe actions a person can take to improve their recovery from surgery. However, it can be applied to any medical treatment that may be needed to treat cancer. It is really a commonsense idea. If you are physically and mentally well prepared for your cancer treatments, then you can expect to be more resilient to the rigours of treatment and any expected (or unexpected) side effects and recover more quickly to resume your preferred lifestyle.

Beyond this, a diagnosis of cancer can serve as a wake-up call to take better care of your health overall, something health professionals like to call a 'teachable moment'. In this way of thinking, the challenges you are facing right now may represent an opportunity to prioritise your health and make lifestyle changes that you might have occasionally considered but not yet acted on.

In general, it is fair to say that many of us, based on global statistics, are not our ideal healthy weight, don't exercise enough, perhaps consume more alcohol than is wise, and report feeling anxious

DOI: 10.4324/9781032638843-3

or stressed more than we should or would like. Some of us may use tobacco products or other unhealthy substances or don't eat a balanced diet. A change towards a more healthy lifestyle can not only support a stronger recovery from cancer treatment but can also improve a person's health in general and contribute to the prevention of other common chronic diseases such as cardiovascular disease.

And yet, even though a diagnosis of cancer might be a teachable moment, our own research has shown that many people do not improve their lifestyle after a diagnosis of cancer, and this likely reflects that changing health habits is not easy. We will have developed our dietary and physical activity habits and our approach to mental wellbeing over many years, and they are well-practised. Changing these, especially when you are unwell and busy managing the practical side of cancer treatments, is not easy. What is important is clarity around what you need to change and a well-thought-out plan. Steps you can take that may help include:

- reviewing your current health status and areas where improvement is needed;
- setting realistic goals for change;
- seeking expert advice on what this change ideally would look like;
- developing strategies for change that are practical for you;
- enlisting support from people close to you in the changes you make.

We suggest starting with changes you feel are most closely aligned with what you value the most or are most concerned about and seek advice from your health care team about what your priority recovery challenges are likely to be.

For example, consider if you need to reduce your weight, or alternatively, if your health care team is more concerned that you maintain your current weight and don't lose condition. There may be specific strategies for different treatment effects that require specialist advice, so ask about these.

Taking action that will help you recover more quickly or respond better to treatment and matching this where you can with behavioural changes that have long been on your 'to do' list is a good place to start.

A final rule, though, is that it is usually easier to learn and change behaviours before you start to feel unwell, so don't wait – get in early!

I AM NOT SURE I AM READY FOR CHANGE: HOW DO I START?

A well-used model that can help here is the Stages of Change model. (1) This model first proposed five key stages: pre-contemplation, contemplation, preparation, action, and maintenance.

If you are in pre-contemplation, then changing or taking up a new behaviour is not yet on your radar. Odds are, though, that your diagnosis of cancer has pushed you into contemplation of making some changes, so now you might be thinking about it. The process of contemplation leads to making a decision. This might be to make a change, to stay the same and not change, or to delay making a change. Chapter 2 about decision making strategies might be helpful to you in your contemplation of possible lifestyle changes. For example, think about your priorities and what matters to you most in the present moment, and then weigh up the pros and cons of making a change.

Once you decide to make a change, preparation is key. This means being clear about what you want to change and what your goal is, planning what steps you will take to make this change along with milestones and a timeline for action, and what resources, advice, and support you will need. Progressive steps that work to a steady build towards your goal often work best.

Action comes next, and while your motivation is high, this may seem like plain sailing, at least for a while. If the plan goes awry, problem-solving and getting 'back on the horse' is the best approach. As you move into maintenance, remember that slip-ups and setbacks are not unusual in any major lifestyle change and that feeling guilty or blaming yourself is not helpful. This is the maintenance stage.

The process of changing our lifestyle is seldom linear. Priorities and circumstances change over time. Try to take a supportive self-coaching approach and recognise small changes as important steps towards where you want to be. Be your own best friend.

EXERCISE MEDICINE: WHAT IS EXERCISE MEDICINE?

For some time now, health professionals and researchers in cancer have recommended that people who have been diagnosed with cancer should avoid physical inactivity and should regularly exercise. The benefits of exercise after cancer include improvements in mood, lower levels of depression and anxiety, less fatigue, and better overall quality of life and physical functioning. (2) Ideally, the type of exercise a person undertakes is prescribed for them to take into account their starting fitness levels, the type of cancer they have, specific treatment side effects, and any limitations they have, such as pre-existing mobility problems or other illnesses.

The effects of exercise for people with cancer go beyond general fitness benefits. The forced inactivity that often goes along with cancer treatments, for example, being in hospital for treatment or having surgery, will cause a loss of fitness and condition in most people. Targeted exercise can help minimise this loss of condition. Some anti-cancer drugs cause muscle or bone density loss and changes in sexual function, to name just a few treatment-specific effects. Prescribed exercise can slow or, in some cases, even reverse these changes.

There is also exciting research going on about a possible anti-cancer effect from exercise. (3) We know from epidemiological data that people who have been diagnosed with cancer who exercise live longer than those with cancer who don't. Researchers have shown that alongside improving body composition and cardiorespiratory fitness, regular exercise can improve immune function and decrease systemic inflammation in the body. Emerging laboratory research also suggests that moderate to high-intensity interval exercise 'snacks' can suppress cancer cell growth. There is a lot to gain from tailored physical activity.

So, what do we mean by exercise? Will a walk in the park do the trick? The World Health Organization advises that adults should do at least 150–300 minutes of moderate-intensity aerobic physical activity, at least 75–150 minutes of vigorous-intensity aerobic physical activity, or a combination of these each week. They also advise muscle-strengthening or resistance exercise at least twice a week. (4) An optimal exercise programme, therefore, includes both aerobic and resistance training.

You will experience more benefits from exercise if it is individualised and planned for you and your specific needs. 'One size fits all' really doesn't work after a cancer diagnosis, tailoring is needed. As well, you are more likely to succeed if your exercise programme is convenient, takes into account your personal circumstances, and includes activities you actually like to do. Some people find they are more motivated if they exercise in a group that might be friends or a local exercise club. Other people prefer to work out on their own.

The best place to start is to talk to your doctor about your planned treatment and then seek a referral to an exercise specialist, such as an accredited exercise physiologist, exercise scientist, or a physiotherapist who has experience working with people with cancer or other chronic diseases. A specialist can help you make a plan that is doable for you and brings the benefits you are looking for. Enlist support from those around you, reward yourself for every gain you make, and notice and enjoy the benefits you experience.

WHAT ABOUT DIET AND NUTRITION?

Your nutritional needs will likely vary during and after cancer treatment. Some people find they gain weight during treatment; others find they lose weight. It is important to ask your doctor what your goals for weight and nutrition should be. Depending on your cancer and the treatment you have had, you might experience changes in your appetite and your sense of taste and smell. Some treatments can cause nausea and vomiting; others can affect the ability to swallow. And when you are tired and stressed, eating a healthy and high-quality diet can seem like another job you simply don't have the energy for.

An accredited practising dietitian can provide individually tailored support and help you plan a diet that will meet your needs and both short and longer-term health goals. Just like for exercise, a personalised (and well-informed) approach will be more effective. Enlisting the support of family and friends is important to help pull it all together and to keep on track. Remember that small changes can make a difference and, over time, get you where you need to be. A good way to move forward with improving your diet is to start by swapping out highly processed foods for more healthy options, one step at a time.

So what are the healthy options? You will often hear that a Mediterranean diet is best for good health, but what does this actually mean? Most guidelines for a healthy lifestyle advise nutrient-dense dietary patterns that include fruits, vegetables, legumes, wholegrain cereals, nuts, and lean meat. (5) Avoiding ultra-processed foods is also recommended. A better-quality diet is associated with better mental health in several studies, although the mechanisms for this are unclear. So there is a lot to gain from improving your diet, even if this is in slow changes.

HOW CAN I MANAGE FEELINGS OF STRESS?

Stress is a normal part of everyday life. Stress can be useful if it motivates us to solve problems or take action that is needed to manage life challenges. The situation to avoid is stress that feels overwhelming or that gets in the way of paying attention to the things and people that most matter to us.

In Chapter 1, we described the stress and coping model, explaining how thoughts, feelings, physiological arousal, and actions interplay to influence how we respond to major life events like a diagnosis of cancer. The usefulness of this model is to see what parts of the stress response we can change to feel more comfortable and in control. In this chapter, we start with physiological arousal, the flight and fight response, and some strategies that may help reduce this response.

Physical activity, as we have outlined earlier in this chapter, is an excellent way to reduce the physiological arousal that we experience as tension or stress and to build up our resilience to stress. In sum, as well as building our physical health and resilience, physical activity can provide mental health benefits and increase feelings of wellbeing.

Other strategies we can learn that directly target the stress response include slow, controlled breathing exercises, progressive relaxation, imagery, meditation, and mindfulness.

An easy breathing exercise is to sit comfortably, lay your hand on your stomach, and then slow your breathing down to a count of four on the in breath and four on the out breath. Your breathing should be deep so that your hand rises as you breathe in. As you do this, focus on the breath and how it feels as air enters and leaves your body. You can extend this exercise by then holding for a count of two after the in breath. Slow breathing is an excellent way to reduce feelings of tension, and a great aspect is that no one needs to know you are doing this. So, if you are feeling anxious while waiting in a doctor's room or anywhere, really, focus on your breath and slow it down.

Mindfulness exercises aim to bring your awareness to the present moment and still a busy mind. This can be as simple as visually focusing on a single point in your environment and looking at this with curiosity and interest or turning your attention to the sounds you can hear around you.

WHAT ABOUT INTEGRATIVE ONCOLOGY?

You may have heard people talking about Integrative Oncology and wondered what this refers to. The definition provided by the Society of Integrative Oncology' is as follows: "a patient-centred, evidence-informed field of cancer care that utilises mind and body practices, natural products, and/or lifestyle modifications from different traditions alongside conventional cancer treatments". (6) Reviews of mind-body therapies have found evidence of improved mood and quality of life from music therapy, meditation and yoga, and relaxation exercises such as guided imagery and progressive muscle relaxation. Tai Chi/Qigong may help with fatigue and insomnia. Hypnosis can be used in preparation for surgery to assist with pain management. (7)

Some cancer treatment centres offer Integrative Oncology, so find out what is available to you and then see how these offerings match up with your personal preference and values.

WHERE DO I FIND SUPPORT?

Having cancer can be a very lonely experience. While those around you might be there for you as much as they can, they are not actually going through this experience. It is a different experience for them standing by, but they can help. Turning outward towards people you trust who are close to you can help reduce feelings of isolation, and these networks can provide a buffer to stress by helping with practical problems, finding useful information, and providing an avenue for you to talk out loud about how you are feeling. Your close social support people and family can also help with encouraging you in any new health habits you are trying out and helping you keep tabs on your progress.

If you do not have a close support network, in many places there are cancer support networks available in the community, such as support groups or peer support programmes where you can talk to someone who has had a similar experience. Some of these groups and networks meet face-to-face, while others connect by telephone, social media, or in facilitated Internet groups. Examples of organisations where you can find these support networks are listed in the Resources and Connections section at the end of this book.

ARE THERE THINGS I NEED TO DO TO PREPARE FOR TREATMENT?

For some treatments, there will be specific actions you need to take to get ready for treatment. For example, for surgery that involves the urinary tract, pelvic floor exercises might be needed in advance of treatment and in the recovery phase to help manage any post-treatment leakage. Physiotherapy support can help here with early recovery of function. If you expect that treatment will cause hair loss, you might want to get ready with hair clippers or organise a wig or hair piece. For some treatments, sexual activity might be affected, so advice from a specialist nurse, sexual therapist, or sexologist might be needed.

Your doctor or treatment team should be able to advise you about what is indicated in your situation and where you can seek advice and support.

HOW DO I KEEP TRACK OF MY CARE PLAN?

Ask your doctor or nurse if they have a survivorship care plan suitable for you. Survivorship care plans usually include details of the cancer treatment plan, side effects to be aware of, follow-up appointments, and strategies to maintain wellbeing. Examples of survivorship care plans that are accessible on the web are included in the *Resources and Connections* section of this book. Some are general, and some are specific to certain types of cancer. Survivorship care plans are designed to be completed in collaboration with your health care team and updated as things change.

JEFF'S REFLECTION

Recently in the 'Lifestyle' supplement of a local newspaper appeared the headline "Are we overcomplicating the Wellness message". Need to keep it simple, too right! I reckon! So I took a look and read that the wellness industry is complicating what should come naturally with attempts to influence choices promoting particular products and services, and so it goes from a consultant psychologist. Who knew? Along with a reminder about individual differences and one size not fitting all, the authors nuzzle it down to three simple things; these are #1 Eating Whole foods, #2 Sleep, and #3 Physical Activity. Really, is that it? Should be straightforward.

Nothing new here. If you Google 'wellbeing', there are thousands of prescriptions and admonishments. There is evidence for beneficial effects on our wellbeing of a balanced/healthy diet, being physically active, and attending to our psychosocial tone. Therein lies the rub. We mostly know the what, question is the how.

Then think cancer.

Nutrition when taste has gone on extended leave to somewhere the cytotoxins aren't. At best, you're feeling bilious, if not straight out nauseous, maybe even with your head in the bowl. Whole foods sure, hard to swallow with the taste of a cereal box. Bring on the chocolate and comfort food.

Sleeping when trying to think away the pain in long bones from GHSF (growth hormone stimulating factor). Trying not to take the prescribed painkillers and sleeping pills, too many pills. Spitting every few minutes from drug-induced excitement of the salivary glands and wrought with worry for wife and children if the remission fails. What were those statistics again?

Movement when the fog of fatigue is an ever-thickening layer of claustrophobia, which suffocates energy and obliterates motivation. Oh, and anyway, it's hard to breathe due to recurrent lung infections, or because of the chemotherapy induced neuropathic pain in feet and hands, or because of the latest blood count numbers, 'make sure you take it easy'. Or being bloated with steroids or any other of numerous disease and treatment impositions.

But are these reasons, or are they excuses? Or something else, like context, within which we have choices to make. Because in the end, no matter where we find ourselves, the responsibility for wellbeing rests with us and how we respond to what is in front of us.

So, for those with recipes for wellbeing, a reminder, just knowing what is good for us, does not always convert to behavioural change, to action. Researchers and clinicians use models to describe this, stages of change for example. A continuum, which we move along one way or another, based on individual and contextual circumstances, pre-contemplation, contemplation . . . and so it goes. Drink less alcohol, exercise more . . . sure, we know, but how do we do it?

The Greek ascetics, think Seneca, believed the denial of physical or psychological desires is necessary to attain spiritual wellbeing. So then, if our physical and psychological desires are denied not through conscious effort but through the ravage of disease, will wellbeing follow?

In the end, each of us needs to work with what is in front of us. Acceptance is in there. What is on the table? What can I change, and what 'just is'? There are choices to make and consequences to balance. And then too, is the matter of what energy, motivation, and angst you have in the tank. To fuel whatever actions you prioritise. Does getting through the day without vomiting come to mind? Important, but so too is the informed and purposeful pursuit of feeling better, being active in your own recuperation, your own health and wellbeing, in whatever direction that takes you. A tip about direction, look inside, heart and soul, for a compass, pointing to the things worth fighting for. There is power there, maybe more than you know.

The best fit for personal wellbeing is grounded in doing the best we can. Do the best you can in whatever the time allowed, no matter if it seems unfair. Shift the focus from what we do not have to what we do have and put that to good use. There are evidence-based recipes, for wellness, find one to suit, tick off the ingredients and get cooking. Mix it up, experiment, and make it yours. Most important is to give it a crack!

Back to ancient Greece, where Seneca and friends applaud quality over quantity: "Life is long enough", we are told, "and it has been given to us in sufficiently generous measure to allow us the accomplishment of the very greatest things if the whole if it is well invested".

For each of us, investing well with what we have is enough. It has to be.

But don't just take my word for it, or that of Seneca's. There is also the wisdom of Lynyrd Skynyrd, from "Simple Man (1973)", in which we are encouraged to take our time and not to live too fast. Troubles will pass. All we need is in our souls if we can only live simply with love and understanding.

So there you have it, all that you need is in your soul. But feel free to eat a healthy diet, sleep well, and exercise; these, too, will help.

SUZANNE'S REFLECTION

When Jeff was having chemotherapy, I was very keen for him to exercise as best he could. Colleagues had told me this would aid the effectiveness of the treatment, and I knew he was losing condition as a result of 'in hospital' activity restrictions, the terrible fatigue he was experiencing, and his loss of appetite and taste. I got busy finding exercise protocols for him and even brought in a new set of resistance bands for resistance training. Alongside this, I did my best to replace the completely abysmal hospital food with what I could source nearby and bring to him each day. Friends were really helpful here in dropping meals off for us periodically.

But, to be honest, while he was in hospital, we had to do our best with stair walking, and we never really got on top of the nutritional challenges. Once I got Jeff home, it was possible to experiment with different foods and start to get back to normal activity, but it has been a long journey. Home was really the best place for him to recover.

Jeff did lose all his hair from his chemotherapy. I was prepared with a good pair of hair clippers so that as soon as this started happening I could keep it very short. It is quite startling to wake up and find your hair in the bed not attached to your head, so keeping it close was helpful in managing this. There were of course other side effects, but we were pretty well-informed and ready for them. They were still awful but we had a plan.

For me as a partner, exercise just went out the door and my eating (and drinking) habits weren't great. There was just too much to do to keep our home going – cattle, chickens, and dogs to feed, yard work to be done, my actual day job, and something had to give. People who cared about me were always telling me to look after my own health as well, but I could not see that as a focus while Jeff was so ill. How did anyone think that was even possible? Now just over two years later I am starting to get back on track with my own fitness with the help of an exercise physiologist and eating better in small steps. It's a work in progress.

REFERENCES

1. Prochaska JO, DiClemente CC. Stages and processes of self-change of smoking: Toward an integrative model of change. Journal of Consulting and Clinical Psychology. 1983;51(3):390–5.

2.   Campbell KL, Winters-Stone KM, Wiskemann J, May AM, Schwartz AL, Courneya KS, et al. Exercise guidelines for cancer survivors: Consensus statement from international multidisciplinary roundtable. Medicine & Science in Sports & Exercise. 2019;51(11):2375–90.

3.   Jenkins DG, Devin JL, Weston KL, Jenkins JG, Skinner TL. Benefits beyond cardiometabolic health: The potential of frequent high intensity 'exercise snacks' to improve outcomes for those living with and beyond cancer. Journal of Physiology. 2023;601(21):4691–7.

4.   World Health Organization. Global action plan on physical activity 2018–2030: More active people for a healthier world. World Health Organization; 2019.

5.   Marx W, Manger SH, Blencowe M, Murray G, Ho FY-Y, Lawn S, et al. Clinical guidelines for the use of lifestyle-based mental health care in major depressive disorder: World Federation of Societies for Biological Psychiatry (WFSBP) and Australasian Society of Lifestyle Medicine (ASLM) taskforce. The World Journal of Biological Psychiatry. 2023;24(5):333–86.

6.   Witt CM, Balneaves LG, Cardoso MJ, Cohen L, Greenlee H, Johnstone P, et al. A comprehensive definition for integrative oncology. Journal of the National Cancer Institute. Monographs. 2017;2017(52).

7.   Carlson LE, Ismaila N, Addington EL, Asher GN, Atreya C, Balneaves LG, et al. Integrative oncology care of symptoms of anxiety and depression in adults with cancer: society for integrative oncology–ASCO guideline. Journal of Clinical Oncology. 2023;41(28):4562–91.

4

HOW DO I KNOW IF I AM COPING WELL?

WHAT DOES *'COPING WELL'* MEAN?

After a diagnosis of cancer, people will often ask how you are coping. That can be hard to answer, and what does 'coping well' really mean anyway? 'Coping' as a term refers to strategies or responses a person applies to a situation in order to manage challenges or struggles. Over the course of our lives pretty much all of us will come across situations or events that are difficult to face, unpleasant, and often unexpected. When this happens we have to pull on our reserves and our skills and strengths to take the actions that are needed and to weather through. Most of us will have developed a style of how we tend to do this and who we call on to help. We learn ways of getting through hard times by watching how other people close to us cope, like our parents or friends, and by seeking advice from people we trust. And experience will have taught us through trial and error what seems to work best for us. Some approaches will be more helpful than others in solving problems or creating a path forward or a sense of ease or control. This chapter talks about what we know about coping from the field of psychology, with the goal of helping you check on your approach, how well this is working for you, and perhaps trying out different strategies.

DOI: 10.4324/9781032638843-4

The general idea here is not that any one approach is necessarily the best. Different situations will likely need different approaches. A way to think about this is that your different ways of coping are like tools in a toolbox; if one tool is not suitable or working for you, being flexible to try a different approach is important. Sticking to one approach for all situations might work some of the time, but probably not all of the time. This is where flexibility comes in.

Psychologists have different ways of looking at 'types' of coping strategies. One approach is to categorise coping as problem, emotion, or meaning-focussed coping. Problem-focussed coping refers to active strategies or behaviours to take action to solve or get through the problem. Emotion-focussed coping covers efforts made to reduce unpleasant emotions, like feeling anxious or sad, that have resulted from a situation of challenge or threat. Meaning-focussed coping is when a person seeks to develop a sense of meaning out of the problem they are facing.

WHAT IS PROBLEM-FOCUSSED COPING?

Studies have shown that problem-solving coping is associated with people feeling less distressed after a cancer diagnosis. Effective problem-solvers are more systematic and have a clearer understanding of the challenges they are facing, and they tend to see challenges or difficulties as problems that can be solved. (1)

The first step in problem solving is to identify clearly what the problem is. This is called problem definition. In order to do this, a person usually needs to seek information about what they are facing from a credible source and get all the relevant facts. You may be facing a number of problems so disentangling them is important, and then prioritising these problems in order of urgency and simplicity. Some problems might be easy to solve once you are clear about the issue, and so sorting these out and getting them off your 'to do' list can create the cognitive space you need to work on more complicated problems. You might even be able to delegate some problems to other people who have offered to help, and again, this gives you some space to direct your attention to where you need it most.

Getting a clear and accurate picture of your most pressing problem is important. When people are anxious, and when they have cancer, feeling anxious is not uncommon, they tend to adopt a more negative perspective that may not represent the actual situation. So, seeking information and talking the issue over with knowledgeable and supportive people can help regain a sense of balance. Sometimes, there can be a chain of problems influencing each other. A good approach then is to pick a place to start that you feel you can influence or most easily have an effect.

Once you are clear about the priority problem to be fixed, you will be better placed to set a goal about what you want to change and exactly how you want things to be different. It is important here to be specific.

The next step, then, is to generate a list of possible actions you might take to move towards that goal, the likely outcome of different actions, and what approaches you feel you have the most resources and energy for. For most actions we take where we want something to change, there will be both costs and benefits. Applying a cost-benefit analysis of different strategies will help you decide on your preferred course of action. This process of weighing up the pros and cons is not unlike the contemplation phase of behaviour change we discussed in Chapter 3. Seek support in your plan from people close to you who can best help.

Once you move into your action plan, regularly evaluate how you are going, be realistic about what change you can expect and when, and be prepared to adjust or reformulate your plan if needed. Again, being flexible is key.

WHAT IS EMOTION-FOCUSSED COPING

Some problems do not lend themselves easily to problem-solving. And sometimes what is needed most is the opportunity to reduce the physical arousal and bodily tension that people can experience in response to the cancer experience or simply express the emotions that might be bottling up.

In Chapter 3, we discussed stress management and lifestyle strategies that can be helpful in reducing stress and building strength. Strategies that directly target the stress response, such as slow controlled breathing exercises, progressive relaxation, imagery, meditation, and mindfulness, can be helpful. Learning these techniques adds additional tools to your coping toolbox.

Physical activity can reduce unpleasant feelings of arousal and improve mood, as well as combating treatment side effects. Activities that involve the connection of physical movement with the outdoors or nature can reduce feelings of tension or distress. This can be as simple as a hike in a forested area or a gardening project that leads to more nature-connectedness. In fact, researchers suggest that a combination of walking or jogging, resistance training, immersing yourself in green spaces, and connecting with other people while doing this together might have the best effect on improving mood. (2) Dancing also has positive effects on mental health!

Connecting to other people on its own can make a difference. Making time for talking with friends or family provides an opportunity to express fears and worries, and often, once these are spoken out loud, they can seem less daunting. Talking over issues can help you to process the situation you are in and develop more of a sense of ease about where you are at, as well.

WHAT IS MEANING-FOCUSSED COPING

First up, you don't need to find a meaning or make a 'good' out of having cancer. It might be that the experience of cancer leads you to reflect on your life priorities, what matters most to you, and where you want to direct your energies in the future. This is a useful consideration for people to make regardless of their health concerns. It is not a job you have to do because you have had a diagnosis of cancer. In Chapter 8, we discuss strategies to consider your deepest values and priorities and how to move towards those in daily life.

Some people find that after having had cancer, they want to give back and help others. This might be through providing peer support to other people having a similar experience, through raising funds for cancer research, or simply getting more involved in community life. This is a great way to build social capital in your community, and there are many not-for-profit cancer control agencies and health services that will value your skills and experience. If this is for you simply reach out to groups around you.

ARE THERE PITFALLS TO BE AWARE OF?

The one coping approach that tends to be mostly unhelpful is avoidance. Avoidance is when you avoid thinking, talking, or considering what is happening, and it is what we might move towards when a situation is emotionally painful. Examples of avoidance are never talking about the cancer or the difficulties you are facing, trying not to think about the cancer and pushing down thoughts about it, or avoiding any reminders of it. In a way, it is closing off your awareness of the present moment. This approach can lead to feeling isolated and cut off from support from others, impede making decisions and solving problems, and over time, the negative emotions and thoughts may become stronger and more difficult to manage. So, while at times, dropping into an avoidant approach might feel right, it is usually not helpful if this is your main or dominant coping method. If you feel you are mostly taking an avoidant approach, you might take some small steps to engage more with what is happening. A good way to start is by making time to talk over the issues with a trusted family member or friend or talking to a health professional about what is worrying you the most. Think of this as putting your toe in the water, testing the temperature, and easing in.

JEFF'S REFLECTION

"Cancer patients are not passive recipients of support". This message is one of the first lessons I learned over decades of working with cancer patients. I cannot recall the source, so

I apologise to the author for my failure to attribute it, but it has stuck with me. The message had a second part along the lines of, "Patients actively seek out those sources of support best suited to their needs and personality", or something like that.

Before I was diagnosed with cancer, I found this sentiment appealing as a frame of reference for understanding the needs, preferences, and behaviours of cancer patients and how to address them. Since being diagnosed, it still rings true, perhaps more so.

Coping with a threat, any threat, is a prime responsibility for individuals, it is central to getting on with life. In every life, there will be threats, and our ability to cope with them determines, to some extent, how each of us fare as individuals. From the most basic fight or flight adrenaline-rush response to more cerebral contemplations about the universe and an individual's place in it, there are as many approaches to coping as there are views on how to go about it and how to gauge success. Google 'coping with cancer', and you will see what I mean.

There are people who fervently believe that every person diagnosed with cancer should, must, attend a support group. Press-gang them outside the Oncology clinic, almost. For others, the thought of attending a support group is anathema. There are others who take every pamphlet, every information sheet, to read and research, that is the answer. Well, not for everyone, it seems. There are those who make sense of the world through talking at it, all the while wrestling, grappling, interrogating, testing, and, in this way, coping with a diagnosis and all that it entails. There are others who by nature and preference, make sense of the world and its multitudinous challenges through internalising and contemplating, quietly and privately bringing to bear the subtle energy found in awareness and acceptance. Each approach and all in-between as preferences evolve are active choices, though to the observer, this may not be apparent.

For me, the message is it doesn't matter what you do, but how you feel about it. There is no simple recipe for success-ful coping. There is a menu from which you can choose, but no recipe. Choose those things to suit your appetite and taste, understanding that these will change over time.

Coping for me was multifaceted. Being cocooned in a close and supportive family, with a devoted and skilful wife as primary carer and cheerleader, was an advantage of incalculable benefit. Acceptance was in the mix, so it goes, as was problem-solving with a focus on making the best choices from options available to me.

Be alert and open to the unexpected as friends, family, and colleagues respond to the news of the diagnosis. Coping can be as much about receiving gifts from others, freely given, as much as it is about personal resources. A tremendous source of support for me arrived quietly and unheralded each day for six months at around 6.00 am in the form of a text message from an old friend. We had been at boarding school together, then at University, I was best man at his wedding, and I am God-father to one of his children. Every morning, I was reminded that there were people out there who cared about my welfare, and I was encouraged to make the best of what the day delivered. It made a difference.

Fight, if that works for you, or quietly seek understand-ing, if that is more to your style. Depend on others, or face it alone, as you prefer. Or any combination in between. To this day, I actively seek out those sources of support that will help me cope, and on occasion, I actively choose to passively accept what is on offer. Some days, I don't. Doing well.

SUZANNE'S REFLECTION

I tend to be a problem-solver in life in general, sometimes a bit too much. A potential misstep for me can be trying to think up the answer before I really know what I am facing. As soon as I see a challenge, I want to work out how to fix it. Over time I have learned that I need to slow this down to make sure I have the full picture and pull myself back to what I actually know rather than imagining what might be to come. As well, problem solving is of course all well and good, but sometimes the problem itself can't be actually fixed by you. What I mean is, for us, the problem we needed to fix was Jeff's cancer, but treating this was the haematologist's job.

So, the problem solving I needed to do was sorting out the medical administrative tasks (that is, all the forms, bookings, and appointments – and there were a lot) and making sure we were on top of all of this. Jeff had to travel for treatment as we were living in a regional area. This meant there was a lot to manage for him as well as accommodation for me to stay in town when Jeff was in hospital. All those things had to be sorted. I had to organise time off work for myself so I could focus on Jeff and the work that needed to be done to allow him to focus on getting well. While I was busy doing jobs, my feelings of distress went on the back burner, just so I could function and get it all done.

Every now and again though I could sense my own feelings of frustration and pain getting stronger, and when this happened I would try to find time to get busy in the paddock feeding the cattle or pulling out weeds just to get physical and focussed on something close to nature. I find being outside and in the natural environment really grounding.

I also had a few close friends that I could call and basically cry with. I think having a safe space to just let your emotions out is helpful. Most of the time I was busy and on top of it but then every now and then I would feel overwhelmed with feelings of sadness, and when that happened, hope seemed hard to visualise and find, just out of my grasp. In the end, I decided I had to let myself feel sad from time to time and then pull myself back into the present moment, whatever that actually looked like. So to let us both have good days and bad days and be okay with that, and bring myself back to the here and now.

Cancer really is for many people a chronic disease and that is a hard reality to face. You or your loved one lives day to day with the physical toll that treatment brings and the uncertainty about what might be ahead. It is tough. In the end, I think you do what you can and then focus on what matters right now and where you can see and feel joy. Dance when you can!

REFERENCES

1. Nezu AM. Helping cancer patients cope: A problem-solving approach. Washington, DC: American Psychological Association; 1998.
2. Noetel M, Sanders T, Gallardo-Gómez D, Taylor P, del Pozo Cruz B, van den Hoek D, et al. Effect of exercise for depression: Systematic review and network meta-analysis of randomised controlled trials. BMJ. 2024;384:e075847.

5

IS THERE A HELPFUL WAY TO THINK WHEN UNDER STRESS?

WHAT IS A THOUGHT ANYWAY?

Cognition or thinking is often described as being a central characteristic of the human condition. The famous philosopher René Descartes referred to this in his famous statement: "I think, therefore I am". This was his first principle – if I can think, I must exist. Human beings have a long history of 'thinking about thinking', and trying to work out what thoughts exactly are, where they come from, and how they might be changed for good or bad.

Scientists tell us that thoughts are formed when nerve cells (or neurons) release chemical messengers (called neurotransmitters) that start a wave of electrical activity in the brain. These waves are our thoughts, a map of what we perceive around us; in a sense, a representation or interpretation of ourselves and our world. This internal interpretation is uniquely our own and guides our response to the external world.

There is an argument that all of our thoughts are unconscious and that our 'inner self-talk' is our interpretation of our unconscious thoughts, guided by our perception of our own internal sensory state and our external environment. (1) For example, our internal sensory state might be one of high arousal or fear and scanning for threats.

DOI: 10.4324/9781032638843-5

Or it might be one of low arousal and feeling calm. We might see our external environment as one of danger or, alternatively, feel safe and secure. From these perceptions we generate a picture of the situation and a pattern of inner self-talk.

Whether we tend to see situations as threatening or manageable might depend at least in part on our past life and experiences as we grew up. For example, if we experienced hard times or felt unsafe growing up, we might tend towards expecting or imagining the worst. If the people around us were mostly worriers, we might have learnt that as safe way of being. In this situation, worrying can almost seem like an action to take to keep safe or a way to divert your attention from the actual problem. (2)

By contrast, if most challenges in our lives were manageable, we might tend to expect problems to be solved and that things will work out in the long run.

The way we think is a very individual thing and not a matter of right or wrong, just individual differences.

So then, why do our patterns of inner self-talk matter? They matter because our inner self-talk guides our view of the world, our situation, and our feelings and influences our responses and actions. Our thought maps can help us, or in the case of excessive worrying, they can exhaust us.

Importantly, this pattern or map of thoughts is not a fact. Rather, our thought map, or inner self-talk, is our *interpretation* of ourselves or our situation, and if it is not helping us, we have a choice.

We can change the interpretation or thought map to be more helpful to us, or we can become less reactive to it.

WHAT ARE SOME COMMON THOUGHT PATTERNS?

There are some common thought patterns that, if they recur and dominate our thinking, can increase and maintain feelings of anxiety and distress. These include:

Catastrophising: Imagining the worst possible outcome and feeling sure this will happen. For example, thinking, "My treatment is sure to fail, and I will definitely get the worst side effects. And then my partner will leave me".

Black and white thinking: Thinking things have to occur one particular way and that if they don't, this is a disaster. For example, "If I don't recover from surgery in exactly eight weeks and get back to my usual life, then I won't ever get better".

Self-blame and guilt: Blaming yourself for everything, for example, "Now I have cancer, I have personally ruined my family's life. Everything is my fault".

Overgeneralising: When one event happens, thinking everything will follow the same pattern. For example, "My blood results weren't good after my first chemotherapy. It will always be like this".

A negative mental filter: This is when we pay attention to the negatives and disregard or don't notice the positives. This can also be called an attentional bias. As an example, dismissing or not noticing positive or stable responses to treatment and instead focussing on what hasn't worked. We tend to have a negative mental filter or lens when we are feeling anxious. It can be a vicious cycle. This is a little similar to *jumping to conclusions*, where we imagine the worst before actually finding out what the situation really is.

It is normal to think in these ways from time to time. But, if these thought patterns are dominating our thinking and we find ourselves ruminating and worrying most of the time, this will increase feelings of anxiety and draw our attention away from things that bring us pleasure or joy. And it is tiring.

A useful first step is to become more aware of your thought maps by reflecting and noticing your thought patterns and how you feel when these thoughts occur. Look at your thinking with interest and curiosity. Perhaps write these thoughts down in a notebook, noting where you were and what you were doing, what was playing over in your mind, and how you were feeling. Where you were and what you were doing will help you identify what might trigger these thoughts. Writing down the thoughts will help you to become consciously aware of your thought map. Noting your thoughts and feelings in this way can help you to understand how your thoughts connect to your emotions or feelings. Once you understand this better, you might decide if this is helping you or hindering you. And if you would like to shift to a place of greater ease in yourself.

CAN A PERSON CHANGE THEIR THOUGHT PATTERNS?

One approach to unhelpful thinking is to decide to change how you are thinking. Not easy for most of us. We will have spent our lives practising certain ways of thinking about the world, and these thinking patterns will be well learnt. It can help to understand where these patterns might have come from and how we learnt to think in this way. But in the end, we need to decide what to do about it and how we want to be right here and right now.

Try to look at your thoughts as objectively as you can and ask yourself if this thought is absolutely 100% true or for certain. Look for evidence about this. Next, ask yourself, 'Is this way of thinking helping me to be how I want to be and do the things that matter to me?' Consider the consequences of carrying this thought map around with you. Ask yourself, is following this train of thought actually going to help me solve the problem or prepare for what is ahead, or does it just feel like it will? Depending on the answer, you can follow the thought or, alternatively, you can challenge it.

To challenge a thought pattern that is not helpful or not absolutely true, try and replace that thought with a different approach that is more balanced. If you had a good friend who was in your situation and thinking in this way, what advice would you give them? Can you become your own best friend?

For example, rather than thinking, "My partner is now burdened by me, and it is all my fault. I have ruined their life". Could you change this to "My cancer is tough for all of us. This is part of life. I didn't choose to get cancer, so it is not my fault. We can support each other through this as a team".

Or, if you experience a treatment setback, rather than thinking, "My treatment is failing, and I have no hope", you could think, "Treatment setbacks are tough and happen. It doesn't necessarily mean a new approach will also fail. My doctor and I can work together on next steps".

The change of a thought map is not denying things are difficult, it is allowing you a way of seeing change in the future as possible and finding hope.

SEPARATING FACT FROM FICTION: WHAT IS COGNITIVE DEFUSION?

A trap many of us fall into is getting caught up in our thoughts and seeming to go round in circles, entangled in our thoughts and over-analysing situations. The outcome of this is usually feeling more anxious and fearful, and our energy is directed into struggling with this rather than the activities that we truly value and that make life feel worthwhile. This is called cognitive fusion, and so the possibility here is to 'defuse' from this unhelpful thinking pattern.

There are a number of different ways to approach this. One is that when you notice you are caught up in a thought 'whirlpool', try and bring yourself back into the present moment, away from worrying about the past or future or what might or might not happen. Present moment awareness can be developed by getting in touch with your senses in this moment. Notice what you can see, hear, and feel around you. Slow down and deepen your breathing, and focus on your breath sensation. Move into the present moment.

Try to put your worrying thoughts to the side for just a few minutes, look at these thoughts with curiosity and some distance rather than sinking into them. If you can, try to imagine your thoughts as sitting in the palm of your outstretched hand, where you can look at them from a distance. Perhaps see this thought map as a pesky critter that has been following you around, but that is separate to who you are. Then, put these thoughts to the side, gently but firmly, and consider whether there is a perspective you might be missing or a different focus for you to pay attention to.

JEFF'S REFLECTION

I often think of the song "Broken Haloes" by Chris Stapleton when I find myself thinking, and thinking, and not seeming to get anywhere. In "Broken Haloes", the general premise is that not everything has an answer, and if it does, it might be a matter best left to the by and by. It's about living in the moment. Having patience. And so, to difficult thoughts!

My wife is a health psychologist and a very good one at that. Happily, there is plenty of free therapy at our house. She often says I need to practice thought-stopping. Unhelpful thoughts no more. Stop them. Full stop. The unhelpful ones that is. Gone.

The reason she "often" tells me to thought–stop is because I can't do it. Not very well. Stopping the unhelpful thoughts is hard. Although she says, "I don't do it", rather than "I can't do it". Like for most things in my life, I am sure she is right, again.

That's the thing about thinking. It just happens, all the time. Thoughts pop up continually, randomly – well, some are random. Others are regulated and rational in response to stimuli and tasks. Complicated.

Factor in a life-threatening disease (AKA cancer) and consequent serious disruptions to important things in your life, and we have fertile ground for unhelpful thoughts. Your thoughts can indeed become interesting, in a Chinese proverb kind of way. Catastrophising, self-blame, if only, imagining the worst, and the list goes on.

Helpful ones and unhelpful ones, all mixed up in a mess of inner-self talk. Thinking about your cancer diagnosis is important, essential, even, and, frankly, unavoidable. There is so much new information, so many unwelcome experiences, and so many changed circumstances; there is a mountain of thinking to do. Where will it end? And when? And why? Always why?

It is how you choose to do your thinking and the focus of that thinking that will lead to one place or another. And no two people are the same about the way they think and the situation in which they find themselves.

Three things.

First, being aware of your thoughts is a mighty first step, a base to begin the difficult task of separating fact from fiction, and so it goes. Some thoughts can be intrusive, and I invite you to put them back in the box.

Second, I am better at thought-stopping than I was. You can practice, and with patience, you can improve, and it does help. Please also take the term thought stopping as a catch-all for any means or method which works for you.

Third, there are ways to think about your own thinking. There are evidenced-based techniques which can help moderate self-talk, focus on issues of therapeutic benefit, and assist in generating a more helpful inner cognitive ecosystem. What are my options, what can I do, and how can this situation be improved? Focussing on things that are more likely to get me where I want to be rather than those that do not is helpful for me.

And it's like exercise; the more you do it, the better you get at being aware of intrusive unhelpful thoughts or self-talk or doubts and stopping them. No time for guilt and shame about why and negative fiction about the future; those things belong to the by and by. I have to invest my time in thinking about getting on with things. That is what I tell myself, just like my wife.

SUZANNE'S REFLECTION

I have a strong problem-solving tendency, and this does tend to keep me focussed on doing rather than thinking. With Jeff's cancer, I have tended to keep my worries to myself and focus on looking for an optimistic bent. In my mind, this is my role as a life partner, supporting him and keeping the ship steady. When I get caught up in a thought pattern of negative 'what if', I try and talk myself down from it by reminding myself that every challenge is a problem to be solved and we will solve it. For example, when our doctor brought up possible future treatments that might be needed, and this was quite scary to even think about, I focussed on getting good advice and generating a game plan. That way I had evidence to combat the 'what if we can't get access to the new therapies' or 'what if the next therapy doesn't work'.

This challenging approach works for me some of the time, especially when the worry is amenable to solving. I will always try this approach first. However, sometimes challenging and problem-solving just leads me into a circular pattern of imagining different scenarios and different ways to solve it and then still ending up back in the same place.

I find the worst time for this is early morning, about 3 am, when I wake up worrying, can't sleep, and can't stop thinking. As the thoughts race around in my head, I can feel the tension in my chest growing. I might feel nauseous, and I am aware my body is reacting as if there is a real and present danger sitting right on top of me. Crushing me. Trying to slow my breathing down and get more grounded physically in the present tends to wind down my stress response a little. And then I wait it out until it passes.

I am still learning to sit with this discomfort and pain when it arises, to treat it as normal and not react to it so strongly or cling to it so tightly. It's about balance, I suppose. In the end, I don't really know what the future exactly holds, but I can influence the present to be the best it can be.

At times, I do think you just have to let the anxiety and fear just 'be' and not pull away from it. In a way, allow yourself to experience it, notice it, and accept it. I find music helps me to sit with my experience and stay with it (my friends tell me I love a dirge). I especially love a cello intro to a song. Then, to move on, I shift my focus to what I can do that engages me physically, like, go for a hike, preferably up a hill, or do something I haven't done before, or for a while. Recently, this was Pilates, which was harder than I remembered!

REFERENCES

1. Carruthers P. The illusion of conscious thought. Journal of Consciousness Studies. 2017;24(9–10):228–52.
2. Verkuil B, Brosschot JF, Gebhardt WA, Thayer JF. When worries make you sick: A review of perseverative cognition, the default stress response and somatic health. Journal of Experimental Psychopathology. 2010;1(1):jep.009110.

6

IDENTITY

WHO AM I NOW?

WHO AM I NOW?

Psychologists suggest that we form our identity through our social interactions, in a process where we identify with others who we see as similar to us and with whom we 'fit'. (1) In doing so, we generate a picture of what personal characteristics, attitudes, and behaviours are important or valuable to us. These characteristics, attitudes, and behaviours then form a map of who we think we are and how we prefer to be, or desire to be, in our world. In other words, our sense of our identity.

A diagnosis of cancer can threaten our sense of self, our physical and mental capacities, and, at a deeper level, who we feel or think we are. If being physically strong and resilient is an important part of your sense of self, then suddenly being physically unwell or weak is not just physically unpleasant; it can rock your self-esteem. Having to hand over or cut back on roles that matter deeply to you can generate a huge sense of loss and grief, for example, if you are not able to work like you used to or care for your family in the same way. Perhaps cancer treatment has changed your sense of who you are as a sexual being and your ability to be sexually close to others the way you were

DOI: 10.4324/9781032638843-6

before the cancer. This can be confronting to a person's identity as a man or woman, and their confidence in intimate relationships may be threatened.

If feeling in control of your present and future is a central part of who you are, then finding yourself in a 'sick role' where the health care team seems to be calling all the shots can feel disorienting and even shocking. Having ongoing medications and treatments can feel like a steep hill to climb, a hill that seems to go on and on, with a constant reminder of the cancer and how life has changed. Changes in appearance, such as hair loss, the loss of a body part, or being constantly fatigued or tired, can be reminders of not being or feeling like the person you were.

As well, misconceptions about cancer and community attitudes, especially with some cancers that can be lifestyle-related, can contribute to feeling damaged or guilty in some way about a diagnosis. For example, people with lung cancer sometimes report experiencing stigma about lung cancer on the basis of this cancer being related to smoking. That it is somehow all their fault, and so they don't deserve help or compassion. This is a very harsh way to be judged or to judge yourself, and people report this experience regardless of whether they were ever a smoker. People who have cancers connected to human papillomavirus (HPV) have described feeling embarrassed about the connection between the virus and sexual activity despite how common HPV infection is globally. What we read or see in the media and the things we hear people say all play a role here.

If a person holds these beliefs or experiences these negative attitudes based on how others respond to them, this becomes an extra burden. If turned inward, this can lead to self-judgement, guilt, and shame, which, in turn, can drive strong feelings of sadness. This is an extra and unfair burden no one needs or deserves.

It is important to say that there is real suffering here. And gripping tightly to what has been lost or has changed can keep us deep in suffering and that sense of loss. Turning toward your experience and finding a different way to look at the situation and a different perspective about yourself that is more flexible can help. We suggest considering five steps:

- Awareness – Become more aware of what the changes in your body and life mean to you and how you are responding to this.
- Acknowledgement – Be your own best friend and give yourself a break. Cancer is tough.
- Present focus – Practice bringing your senses back to the present moment. The present moment is the only thing we know for sure.
- Flexibility – Is there a different way of looking at your present state of being?
- Turning towards – Can you try a different way of responding to where you are now?

WHERE DO I START?

A good place to start is to reflect on what has changed in your life and what this change means to you. You may have been so busy gathering information, making decisions, and getting on with treatment that you haven't found the time or energy to think about yourself in this way. Set aside some time to write this down, and then, over a week or two, reflect back and consider all the changes in your life since your cancer diagnosis; which have been the most difficult? What words would you use to describe these changes? How do you feel physically when you think about this? Try to sit with any feelings of unease and see if you can find some words to describe what this change means to you.

WHERE DOES ACKNOWLEDGEMENT FIT IN?

Naming a loss can be a first step to developing a new perspective about that loss. Can you call this out in some way? Some changes may seem like a heavy load you are carrying or a monkey clinging to your back. Other changes might be more like a bump on the road that you feel you can't get past. Acknowledge what is painful and allow yourself to feel whatever emotions come up. Comfort yourself as you would comfort a best friend or loved one going through the same experience.

HOW DO I FIND PRESENT FOCUS?

Practice drawing your attention to the present moment, especially when you find yourself experiencing strong emotions around the changes in your body and your life since the cancer. Can you notice what you can see and hear around you, paying attention to the details of your surroundings with your sense of sight and hearing? Don't miss the details. Allow any difficult thoughts and emotions to come and go, ebb and flow, all the while gently drawing your attention to what is around you.

WHAT DOES FLEXIBILITY MEAN?

Try to imagine a different perspective or viewpoint you might take about the changes you have experienced and how you see yourself now. Is there a different way of looking at your situation? For example, if you have experienced sexual changes from treatment, is it possible that there is a new way you can express, experience, and show closeness and intimacy with your partner? If your body has changed, you might find a different way of seeing yourself, perhaps as a survivor with scars that are a badge of your courage in facing cancer.

HOW DO I TURN TOWARDS MY EXPERIENCE?

Rather than avoiding your experience, a different approach is to find a new way of expressing who you are and consider in a playful and creative way who you might be next. This might include leaning in to consider the changes in your life with a sense of curiosity and kindness. When you look at the changes in your life in an unguarded way (without the bracing), you might find you are able to shift your perspective on what you see. To start to see yourself as more than the loss and focus more on the whole. Knowing that your essential inner and valuable self remains might free you up to try different strategies. For example, if there are physical pastimes that are now hard to do, there might be small steps towards that activity that you might take. And these small steps are to be savoured. In your relationships and social networks, this might mean finding new ways of connecting and expressing love and friendship. The central idea is not to close down but instead to open up to possibilities.

OUR COMMON HUMANITY

Many of us have a tendency to judge ourselves harshly, and there is an extent to which the environment we live in may encourage or lead us towards this way of thinking. We all have strengths and weaknesses and things we wish we had done differently. We all age, and alongside this, our physical self changes, and we all have a desire to be loved. This is our common humanity. No one deserves to get cancer or should feel guilty about it. We are all worthy. Everyone deserves help and care.

The task here is to be compassionate to ourselves, turn inwards with softness and care, and think of ways we can nourish ourselves in the present, not held back by the past.

JEFF'S REFLECTION

"Cogito, ergo Sum", meaning, "I think, therefore, I am".

Coined by Renee Descartes in the 1600s, this saying highlights the importance of reason and rational thought as confirmation of our existence. At the time, it was a counterpoint to the quotidian grind of feudal drudgery. A noble thought, at once seeking to elevate, to attribute free will, and to challenge assumptions because we can. An identity based on being, on how we think about ourselves.

It has been said that a diagnosis of cancer is a threat to identity, or if not, at the very least, will change how we think about ourselves as individuals.

So, how would Renee codify a cancer diagnosis? I gave it a go with a few things that came to mind and compiled what is, by no means, a comprehensive list. Apologies in advance to Latin scholars (and Renee) for errors in translation/application.

Lucito, ergo Sum – I struggle, therefore, I am.
Spero, ergo Sum – I hope, therefore, I am.
Puguo, ergo Sum – I fight, therefore, I am.
Ego, ergo Sum – I cope, therefore, I am.
Superstes, ergo Sum – I survive, therefore, I am.

How we think about ourselves, the way we are viewed by the world, and the characteristics that define us – some say this is what defines our identity, and if it is, then for sure and for certain, it will change after a diagnosis of cancer. The hope, the coping, and the surviving will affect how we feel about ourselves and how we feel about the world around us, as well as how others see us, judge us, and compare to us. Nevertheless, how we let the disease define us, well, that is up to us.

A cancer diagnosis is a major life threat – of course it will change us. Organisational psychologists confirm that when faced with change, most people focus on the negatives with fear of the possible consequences. There are others, however, who look for the potential, embrace it, and fold it into a new reality, one that is rational under the changed circumstances.

Be yourself, whatever characteristics, conceptions, and interests that this entails, and as far as possible, embrace the change. Accept, mould, and massage the newness and threat and work it into a version of you that is not better or worse than before the diagnosis but that is fit for purpose after. "Knowing yourself is the beginning of all wisdom" (Aristotle), and is there a better way to get to know yourself than facing adversity? Because remember, now and forever, it is not possible for you to be a person who has not had cancer. Character building, as they say! From someone who knows something about adversity: "Character cannot be developed in ease and quiet" (Helen Keller), and after a cancer diagnosis, we definitely have a lack of ease and absence of quiet, so let's make the most of it. Look at yourself, understand and like what you see, particularly the bits which have changed.

I do identify as a person with cancer, but cancer is not my identity. Chip Taylor, singer, songwriter, activist, and also famous for being Angeline Jolie's uncle, offers insight and what I believe to be good advice. In his album, "The Little Prayers Trilogy", there is a song entitled "I'll only be me once". The point is that since we only have one chance to be ourselves, we had better find out who we are.

To borrow from Renee one more time:

"Ergo sum me, ergo sum" – "I am me, therefore, I am". Now there is a thought!

SUZANNE'S REFLECTION

My perception of the challenges for Jeff here related to the physical changes he has experienced from his treatment, especially the fatigue, and secondly, the constant medication and ongoing medical treatment that will not ever stop.

Jeff has been a scarily strong and healthy man, a trekker, never on any regular medication, with a slow, steady pulse, low blood pressure, and fabulous lung capacity, not someone who sees a lot of doctors or who takes pills. So, ongoing intense medical treatment is like a new alien world for him.

The acute treatment phase is a bit of a blur because so much is going on, and it is all very risky and life threatening. But then, after that part is done, the long haul starts. This cancer really is a chronic disease. I think to be thrust into this so quickly is a bit shocking. This almost marks the start of redefining expectations and goals for Jeff as a man and for us as a couple. It is an ongoing process of adjustment with new challenges that emerge over time.

Alongside this, of course, there are the changes that come with ageing, and we both have these. I can certainly talk about that from my perspective as a woman. One of my granddaughters recently pointed her little finger at me and said, "Grandma, you are really old!". And I guess, at least from her viewpoint, I am. As you age, your metabolism slows, you put more weight on around your middle (central adiposity), you lose muscle mass, the wrinkles increase, the grey hair, you are not as agile or quick on your feet, and you are prone to a whole lot of new maladies. It's a lot.

On the other hand, you have wisdom from life experience, and you are still around to enjoy people, family and friends, your favourite pastimes, and the natural environment. It does require a rethink at some point about who you are now and who you want to be in this life transition.

Thinking deeply about your values is important, and trying to pay service to these in your everyday life. It is important to decide where you want to put your energies and what you want to leave behind. This is also a time when you can be a bit playful and creative and give yourself space to try different things (buy that crazy denim jacket, hoop earrings, and let that grey hair grow long and free) and explore different ways of being. So that is where I am now, slowly venturing into new habits and a different self but keeping close to what matters most to me.

REFERENCE

1. Stets JE, Burke PJ. Identity theory and social identity theory. Social Psychology Quarterly. 2000;63(3):224–37.

7

HOW DOES CANCER AFFECT RELATIONSHIPS?

When a person is diagnosed with cancer, there are ripple effects. Family members, partners, close friends, and colleagues may all experience feelings of shock and distress, often alongside feelings of helplessness. Put simply, a person's diagnosis affects the people around them (albeit to varying degrees), and sometimes, it can feel like managing the reactions of other people is another job or burden the person with cancer has to face.

Early questions to think through are: Who do I tell? And then, What do I say? It is a good idea to think this through and decide on a plan. You can always change that plan as needed. But considered and thoughtful communication about how you will approach this with family, friends, and colleagues is more likely to get you the support you need and help you and your close friends or family cope together as a team.

FAMILY

People often worry about telling their children, especially if they are young or at a vulnerable stage in their lives. It is important, though, to be aware that children will often intuit that something is wrong from seeing the people around them looking distressed, talking or

DOI: 10.4324/9781032638843-7

behaving differently, or coming and going in a different way or pace. So they know something is up, and if they don't know the truth, they might imagine something worse or imagine they did something wrong.

Being honest with children can prevent misunderstandings and help them learn how to cope with difficulties in a proactive way by watching you. This is an opportunity for them to learn about life's challenges and develop resilience. Some good basic rules with children are to talk to them at a level appropriate for their age and let their school or close networks know what is going on so that they can work together with you to support your child. Try to schedule activities that are fun and recreational for your children so that life is not just about the cancer. Friends and family might be able to help here. It is also important for parents or caregivers to regularly check in with their children and ask them how they are feeling, check their understanding of what is happening with the cancer (especially if things have changed), and ask if they have any questions. Choose times to talk when things are relatively calm and there are fewer distractions, for example, driving in the car or going for a walk.

Tell your children that you love them. Often.

FRIENDS

The extent to which you wish to let your other social networks know about the cancer is up to you. Having close friends in the loop can be helpful for practical and emotional support and provide you with a more objective listener when you need to bounce ideas around or express difficult emotions. Be clear with friends about how they can help or support you, mostly they will value that advice.

In general, people mean well, however, their own anxiety or fear might lead them to be excessively chirpy or cheerful, seeming to minimise what you are going through. Unsolicited medical advice and stories from past experiences that are not relevant to you can be intensely annoying. Gently letting people know what is not helpful and then what you would prefer can provide guidance that helps all concerned.

Keep a note of all those people who have offered to help just in case you need them in the future. Consider what type of help they might offer that you would find useful. For example, the person you ask to walk your dog may not be someone you would choose to drive you home from chemotherapy or keep you company when you are feeling unwell.

WORK

If your treatment or support of your loved one is going to require some time off work, then talking to your employer about this will likely be needed. As well, after some treatments, a slow or graded return to work might need to be negotiated. Many workplaces have employee assistance programmes that provide free counselling and support, so see if this is available for you. Be aware of your entitlements as a worker for leave and workplace support so that you can plan how to manage any time off work you may need. As far as possible, make sure you take the time off work that you need to heal and recover. This is a time in your life when your health needs to be your priority.

COUPLE RELATIONSHIPS

If you are in an emotionally intimate relationship with another person, a husband, wife, or partner, then you might be wondering about how they will cope with the cancer diagnosis and what changes cancer might bring to your lives as a couple. In general, what seems to matter in this situation is for both of you to be on the same page in how you approach the challenges now and in the future. This means both being well informed about the situation and the challenges ahead and, as far as possible, making decisions together about how you will manage the next steps.

A partner can be a great support in a medical consultation. This gives you an extra pair of ears, someone to take notes and ask questions you might not have thought of, a different perspective to consider, and, in the end, someone else who can help carry the load.

This is not always easy. Your partner may already be under stress through other family or work responsibilities. They might have their own health concerns to deal with. And if you are in a new relationship, you might both still be learning about each other and in the process of building your life together.

As individuals, you will each have your own approach to coping with difficulty, and as a couple, you might also have an already well-established pattern of how you do things. It is likely to help if you can talk over together how you want to approach the diagnosis and treatment and how you think you might help and support each other as you learn to live with this changed reality.

This does not mean you have to talk about the cancer all the time. It does mean, though, that it will help if periodically you take time to talk over your different perspectives, check how the other person is going, and share with each other what you might be able to do differently, or more or less often, to support each other. Sharing how you are going and feeling can also help you not to mind read what is happening for the other person, which prevents misunderstandings.

If you find you are both feeling more tense and anxious than usual, accept that this is not surprising given the situation in which you find yourselves, and try to avoid blaming. Conflict is normal in relationships, and, over time, couples will have developed a style for how they manage conflict. Some approaches are more helpful than others in de-escalating the issue.

A suggested approach is to lead into the issue gently and to try and keep levels of physiological arousal (the fight and flight response) low. (1) Remember that cancer is stressful, so you are both under pressure. Try to stand back from the situation, take a deep, slow breath, and look for a different way forward or a different perspective. Avoid blaming, and as much as you can, show affection for the other person through acceptance and calm. Not everything can, or needs, to be solved and agreed upon. Difference is okay.

WHAT MAKES A HEALTHY RELATIONSHIP?

Experts in couples therapy and self-help suggest different approaches, even some strategies that are known through careful research to be unhelpful. So, buyer beware.

There is though good evidence to support the idea that a sound couple relationship is one where each person is open to and understands the other person's view on life. Strong couple relationships are built by purposeful actions to share each other's world and having shared meaning about what matters most to them. (2) In short, shared values and a commitment to a life together, come what may. Cancer, in many ways, is the 'come what may' that can provide a moment to decide not to sweat the little things so much, forgive and let go of past grievances, and truly have each other's backs.

WHAT ABOUT SEX?

Cancer treatments often affect a person's sexual life. The exact nature of these effects will depend on the type of cancer you or your loved one had and the type of treatment. Being informed about this with advice from your cancer treatment doctor or nurse is important. Ask questions about what you might expect to change and then what can be done to help you restore this aspect of your life. It might feel uncomfortable to talk about this with a health professional, but remember this is their regular job, to educate and inform you about possible or likely sexual changes so you can be prepared and take the necessary actions.

So even if you feel hesitant or a little embarrassed, remind yourself that not knowing and not taking steps towards sexual recovery may needlessly stop an enjoyable and enriching sexual life. If the way you have sex needs to change because of treatment effects, then try to be playful and open minded about new possibilities.

Remember that sexual intimacy is built on emotional intimacy. Keeping the foundation of your relationship strong with love and affection and valued time together will lay the basis for sexual recovery.

JEFF'S REFLECTION

I am a fan of Taylor Swift. A Swifty. Not weird at all for a Baby Boomer (though my adult children think so), as half of her fan base is over 45 years of age, and 25% are Boomers. Who would have thought? She wrote a song, "Soon you'll Get Better" (2019 Lover Album), and the chorus insists you must get better soon, basically just because you have to.

Apparently, she wrote this song after a family member's diagnosis of cancer. The last line resonates for me, the emphatic lament: you need to get better, for yourself sure, but for us too, those of us around you. We need you to get better. You must, you have to!

Prior to diagnosis I had always understood the notion of the ripple effect cancer can have; post-diagnosis, I feel it personally and powerfully. Partners, families, friends, colleagues, workplaces, and whole communities can be impacted by a person's cancer diagnosis, and it can influence and change relationships.

There is a reciprocity here. We love and care for you, and you have to get better. We need you to get better, and as a patient, this realisation serves as a prime source of responsibility and motivation. Reminds me of entry level subjects in the sociology of health where the notion of sick and dying 'roles' are explored. As a society, we forgive an individual who is sick from doing certain duties (work and family commitments, for example) in exchange for that person taking reasonable steps to get better, such as seeking medical advice, complying with treatment, and the like. Fail to do this, and there are sanctions. So for the patients out there, if you thought a cancer diagnosis was all about you, think again. 'Cause having cancer is not just about you! It is also about people around you who have expectations of you, hopes, and, like you, feel bereaved and fearful of an unwelcome alternative future, one where your role and your presence and their life, too, will be different. Of course, it may come to pass that this future is joyful and fulfilling, but who is to know, one way or another? As a patient, you too become a carer for those who care for you. Counter-intuitive, the patient as carer idea, but there it is.

The stress of a diagnosis will have an impact on relationships, depending on the type of cancer, treatment, and prognosis. Strong, loving relationships may evolve and change in ways that are enhancing. Whereas arrangements of convenience based on transactional undertakings, whether formal or unspoken, may suffer as the ability of one partner to uphold their end is degraded financially, physically or socially. Or maybe not. Depends on the actors, the circumstances, and what is at stake. For me, I found the diagnosis and subsequent rigours of treatment served to enrich and strengthen my relationships with family, friends, and colleagues. I am grateful for that.

Back to Taylor Swift's song where, in one verse, she regrets making it all about her, but wonders what to do and who to talk to if there is no you.

There it is, again, as a patient, we have a job to do. Get better "cause we have to" people are depending on us to do so. Selfish, not at all, just human.

SUZANNE'S REFLECTION

When we got the news about Jeff's diagnosis, the first people we needed to tell were our four adult children, aged in their twenties to early thirties. Jeff and I decided together that I would call each of them, be honest about the situation, and promise them that I would keep them all fully informed and as involved in Jeff's treatment and care as they wished to be. These were very hard calls to make, and there were lots of tears, but we set things up as we wanted them to continue. To cope together as a family.

For the more extended family, I called key people and asked them to tell other family members. I really didn't want to make all those calls. I had to let my work know as I needed time off to support Jeff, and they were all wonderful in giving me space while knowing if I needed help, I could reach out. Some colleagues who had some similar experiences were particularly helpful, and are still there now when I need them.

Life after cancer as a couple has an added complexity to it. Jeff has ongoing treatment that requires regular hospitalisation, and the side effects of treatment are harsh. So life changes in many practical ways. I think as a couple we have very solid shared values around family, and, in particular, the importance of the wellbeing and future of our children and grandchildren is central to us. So this goes into all our planning about the future. As well, we both enjoy similar simple pleasures like gardening, planning meals, quality Kentucky bourbon, seeing close friends, and getting out of the city. We prioritise these things and increasingly are saying no to activities (usually fancy events) that don't fit what we enjoy most.

Fitness and health matter to us both, and we support each other in our goals here. We both have busy work lives, but here again, increasingly over time, we are drawing our work focus closer to our shared goals of improving cancer outcomes in our community.

Like any couple, we have disagreements, and we do our best to keep calm and get past them. You don't have to solve everything, some things can't be changed or solved. And you don't have to agree about everything. Life is finite, and there is no time to waste. I try to keep my head up and focus on the main game, the things that really matter to me and Jeff. When we married, I said at our wedding, "Jeff holds my heart in his hand." Still true.

REFERENCES

1. Gottman JS, Gottman JS. Fight right: How successful couples turn conflict into connection. Penguin Books Limited; 2024.
2. Gottman JS, Abrams D, Gottman JS, Abrams RC. Eight dates: To keep your relationship happy, thriving and lasting. Penguin Books, Limited; 2019.

8

I FEEL STUCK

HOW CAN I CHANGE THIS?

LIFE STORIES

In life, we all have our stories. About how we grew up, the good and bad things that have happened to us, the people who helped and the people who hindered, the things we are proud of, and what we might regret. Woven together, this becomes our story or *narrative* about who we are, how our life generally plays out, what we hope for, what we strive for, what we expect, and what we need to live.

Sometimes, though, life throws us a curveball, we find the narrative we have been working with doesn't seem to help us, and we can't seem to move forward or get over the speed bump. In other words, we get stuck. If you are feeling 'stuck' this might mean that you need a different approach to how you are looking at your cancer diagnosis, your future, and how you sit in the world. This counts for people with cancer and their partners equally.

Perhaps you are feeling anxious a lot of the time and are finding it hard to relax and feel easy in your skin. You might be living with a sense of grief and loss that is weighing you down, or worrying a lot of the time about the future and what it could hold. Maybe you are angry or annoyed more than you would like or feel that your relationships

DOI: 10.4324/9781032638843-8

are not working as well as they might. These two things might be linked or closely connected. Or you might be feeling a need for more direction in your life or a shift to a different purpose.

The place to start is with awareness.

WHERE ARE YOU NOW?

Awareness is about taking time to reflect on your story or narrative – how you got to this point in life and what that narrative means to you. Doing the same thing repeatedly will generally lead to the same outcome. Is your current approach serving you well? Are you up for considering change?

To start to think this through set aside some time when you won't be interrupted. Find a comfortable place to sit where your body is well supported and relaxed. Start by building awareness of your breath. Gently place your hands on your belly. If you feel relaxed to do so, close your eyes. Breathe slowly to a count of four for each in-breath and each out-breath. Notice the breath coming into your body through your nose and the temperature of the air as you draw this into your body. Notice how your belly expands as you breathe in and relaxes back as you breathe out. Maintain this focus on your breath and direct your attention to this sensation.

Now start to notice other parts of your body and how they feel. The soles of your feet and what they are placed upon, the pressure you feel there. Notice your posture and whether it is tight or loose. Gently move your shoulders and check for tension in your neck. Notice how your facial muscles are feeling, is your brow relaxed? Is your jaw tight or loose?

As you are doing this, your mind might wander to the worries of the day or the jobs and tasks you have to do and that are on your mind. Notice these thoughts and the feelings that come with them, and how these thoughts affect your body tension. These thoughts and feelings are not in and of themselves good or bad. They just are what they are. Notice them, be aware of them, and now gently direct your attention back to your breath.

Now, listen to the sounds you can hear around you. This might be traffic noises, birds, wind in the trees, or household noises. This is where you are right now, in the present.

So, now, in the present moment, turn to your heart and your head. What changes are you looking for in how you sit in the present? What would this mean for you? What words describe how this would look and feel?

When you are ready, focus again on counting in for four and out for four on each breath, and then open your eyes and jot down the feelings and thoughts you became aware of, and think about these thoughts as if they were a story you have been telling yourself for a long time. The question to ask yourself is whether this story is helping you to live closely to what matters in your life. If you were to change this story, what might that look like now and in the future?

ARE YOU UP FOR A CHANGE?

Next, you need to decide if you are really up for change, what that might mean, and what yearnings or past grievances you might need to let go of. How we live is up to all of us. Life will have delivered highs and lows, successes and losses. Rarely is this all good or all bad. It is our rich tapestry, our story or narrative, and we can become fused or glued to the past and our expectations of the future as if it is the only possible reality. We can get stuck in our past thoughts, feelings, and behaviours, and our expectations that this is all there is or can be. But how you experience the world and those around you *can* change into the future.

Dwelling on the past is not likely to lead to change. Living in the present can lessen the burden of the past, and deciding to make changes for the future brings with it possibilities. No one is perfect, none of us. So accepting that and letting go of 'what ifs' and 'I should have' or 'might have' can be very freeing.

This is about opening up to possibilities, dropping self-blame, suspending judgement of ourselves and those around us, and responding to what we see and experience in new ways. Small changes can make important differences in how closely we connect with people who are important to us and in how we walk into the future with ourselves in a spirit of self-compassion – being the self that we want to be, connecting with others the way we want to.

TRYING OUT CHANGE

Change is hard. Most of us tend to avoid it. A good place to start is to think of some small steps or actions towards how you want your life to be and set yourself up with these as experiments you can try. This is about a pivot to what matters to you most now. For example, if you have relationships that you would like to deepen and appreciate more, think about what you might do differently to move towards this way of being. If wellbeing and fitness are areas you would like to improve, contact an exercise specialist who can advise and support you in making changes. What strategies could you commit to for relaxation, for example, listening again to the music you most loved in your younger years or enjoying a good movie. Look for a short course on a topic you have always wanted to know more about. Perhaps there are activities you have always felt would be fun and rewarding but that you have avoided because of embarrassment or fear or never managing to find the time. Maybe you haven't felt you had earned the chance for change or something new or better. Now is a chance for change where you get a free pass.

Make a list of things you have always wanted to try, and select five to start with. Map out some steps you could take to move towards these new actions and who could help or support you. Schedule each of these activities to try out over the next six weeks. Commit yourself 100% to the effort. No self-evaluation or criticism is allowed. This is an experiment for you in widening out your range and view of what is possible in your life. It's staying with the plan that matters most. Think of this as an opportunity to try acting and feeling differently. Lean in. Try saying yes.

JEFF'S REFLECTION

"The Boy and the Filberts"
A BOY put his hand into a pitcher full of filberts. He grasped
as many as he could possibly hold, but when he tried to pull out
his hand, he was prevented from doing so by the neck of the
pitcher. Unwilling to lose his filberts and yet unable to
withdraw his hand, he burst into tears and bitterly lamented his
disappointment. A bystander said to him, "Be satisfied with half
the quantity, and you will readily draw out your hand".
Aesop Fable

How about life! Full of ups and downs, highs and lows.
Whether you have cancer or not. Pace and tempo evolve, a
rhythm develops, undulates, and while not always comfortable,
it is generally recognisable and serves as a base from which to
get on with the business of getting on with life.

Though, occasionally, we get stuck. Like in a rut. People
diagnosed and treated for cancer may face additional burdens,
making it easier to get stuck. Or get stuck for longer, or find
it harder to get unstuck. Maybe even resign oneself to perma-
nent stuck-ness. The 'living with cancer' rhythm is new and
unrecognisable. The usual reference points and motivators have
changed: which way, which way? Who wouldn't get stuck?

The moral to the "Boy and the Filberts" Fable is to be satisfied with what you have, with what you can do, and try not
to bite off too much at once. Let's agree that slowing down,
easing back from time to time, can be a good thing. So, are
you really stuck or just taking a rest? Recovering from and
coping with cancer does not happen in a neat, straight line at
constant velocity from the point of diagnosis. Be gentle with
yourself.

If you can, sort out what is important and direct your focus there. This is much more likely to motivate. Break it down, bite size. Grand plans and fantasy gestures are fine, but small steps, little gains, one after another, can get you there. More likely to succeed. Set goals if you wish, it works for some, but make them realistic, with a direct line of sight to success. This will help avoid the self-recrimination that is consequent to repeated failure, which is more likely when over-ambitious.

Patience it is said is a virtue, and in this context, I agree. I learnt to be accepting of setbacks. Physical activity is important to me, and I was eager to resume this lifetime habit for mental health as much as physical reasons. However, I was routinely thwarted by side effects of treatment as well as self-inflicted reversals from overdoing it. Too much too soon. I had to recalibrate, take time, more than I would like, and take smaller steps. Patience and discipline. I needed more patience, and discipline, and smaller steps.

There is a book by Kelli Chevalier (2006) titled *Get up, Get dressed and Get out*. Focusing on people struggling with trauma and their mental health, the author offers this simple recipe for transitioning from a life of self-pity to one of purpose. A diagnosis of cancer is a traumatic event, and we know from evidence and personal experience it has an impact on our psychosocial health. No wonder we sometimes get stuck. I did. Still do. I found this simple message, which speaks to sequential bite size tasks, helpful. Clearly others have found it helpful too, for example I found that it has been adapted to 'Get up, Get Dressed and Get Moving', where investigations confirmed patients who do this have better outcomes than those who remain in bed.

Simple message. Uncomplicated. Maybe it will work for you too.

I like reading fables. Wisdom in nugget form. Brief and easy to digest. Aesop's fables feature animals and activities of daily life, with the message compelling but not always apparent; even better. Gets me thinking about things differently, from angles otherwise unnoticed. A reading list for you, a Fable guide to being un-stuck:

"The Tortoise and the Hare" – Never give up.
"The Crow and the Pitcher" – There is always a way.
"The Bell and the Cat" – Ideas are easy; avoid impossible remedies.
"The Hart and the Hunter" – We may despise what is most useful to us.
"The Dog and the Shadow" – Be content with what you have.

There are over 700 Aesop Fables, so plenty to choose from. Let's finish with the "Crow and the Pitcher":

A thirsty Crow comes across a pitcher which had been full of water. But when he puts his beak into the mouth of the pitcher, he cannot reach the water. He keeps trying but then gives up. At last, he comes up with an idea. He keeps dropping pebbles into the pitcher. Soon, the water rises up to the top, and he is able to quench his thirst.

There is always a way. Look for the pebbles, they are all around, friends, resources, professionals, books, nature, whatever; fill your pitcher, bit by bit. Drink deeply.

SUZANNE'S REFLECTION

I have always tended towards trying to live in the service of what matters to me most. Some of this is a constant, for example, our children, our grandchildren, and, of course, my relationship with Jeff. The people closest to me who deserve to get the best of me. This includes my dearest friends and extended family.

It can be a struggle, though. In action, what this means is when I am with those people closest to me, I need to be present and focus on them and what they need, rather than the chatter in my head. This I think is where awareness and being consciously present really matters. We might think we do this, but unless we check, there is always a good chance we are on automatic pilot. And automatic pilot is not being truly present for others.

The same principles apply also to my work. Doing the best job I can for my Faculty staff and the University is important to me, and an absolute priority is being the best therapist I can be for the patients I see. And constantly learning about ways I can do these things better: improving my skills, seeking and taking advice and wise counsel, looking for alternative perspectives, and not being closed off to possibilities.

In all of this, as a partner of a man who has had some pretty rough cancer treatment and has ongoing treatment and side effects from this treatment, it is easy to forget to look after your own wellness. And keeping yourself well is essential in order to be a good carer, if for no other reason.

So, I have started working on a plan to get fit, lose a bit of weight, and improve my flexibility and strength. It is slow going and takes commitment, but it does feel good when you find you can lift a bale of hay with more ease and toss the grandkids around in play without pulling a muscle! And you fall over less!

9

WHAT ARE THE WELLBEING ESSENTIALS?

WHAT DO WE MEAN BY WELLBEING?

Wellbeing is not about the presence or absence of illness or disease. Wellbeing is about the quality of a person's life taking into account physical, emotional, sexual, social, and spiritual aspects of life. It also includes satisfaction with life and happiness. Really, all aspects of life that bring one a sense of *feeling well*. And you will have specific aspects of life and your own priorities that are uniquely important to you for your sense of feeling well. All of us define for ourselves what matters for us most as individuals, what is essential in order to feel well.

A cancer diagnosis threatens our wellbeing across many different aspects of life quality, and it can be a confusing experience. In working with experts who work in cancer and talking to people who have experienced cancer, we have developed a Wellbeing Essentials Framework that provides a map or guide for actions you can take to support your own wellbeing. While we originally developed this for people diagnosed with cancer (1), this framework or map is relevant for any illness or health challenge, especially one that requires ongoing treatment. It is a set of principles you can apply in setting goals for recovery and building and maintaining your wellbeing now and into the future.

DOI: 10.4324/9781032638843-9

WHAT ARE THE WELLBEING ESSENTIALS?

There are six key aspects of wellbeing that are essential in building wellness after cancer. These are:

- Personal Agency
- Values-based Management
- Vigilance
- Teamwork
- Strategies that work
- Finding Meaning

So what does this all mean?

PERSONAL AGENCY

Personal agency is feeling able to influence your wellbeing and being ready (or getting ready) to take actions to improve or maintain your wellbeing in the areas of life that matter most to you. Start with doing a check on different aspects of your quality of life, reflect on what matters to your most, and from this consider what might be your goals for change. Chapter Three in this book talked about contemplating change and getting ready for action – personal agency is your driver to move in this direction.

Personal agency does not mean going it alone. It means utilising all the supports available to you, including your family, friends, and your health care team. Finding out who can help, what you can do yourself, and what others can offer puts you in a position to make decisions about your wellbeing and then, step by step, move forward at your preferred pace.

WHAT CAN I DO?

Set wellbeing goals that most matter to you. In thinking of the months and years ahead, what would you like to work towards? How would you like things to be different in one month, in three months, in a year? You might have some short term goals around managing treatment side effects or more medium term goals about building your physical strength and resilience or feeling more comfortable emotionally and more relaxed in your skin. Strengthening your intimate relationship or perhaps looking to develop one might be on your list.

Once you have your goals clear, you can identify the information and other support you might need to achieve these goals. Set targets that are achievable and put an action plan in place with a timeline. Be prepared to be flexible and problem solve as you go along. This approach will help you to feel more in control of your wellbeing and the plan going forward. Personal agency doesn't mean everything has to be or will be perfect. It is about influencing what is going on and getting some control over the story.

VALUES-BASED MANAGEMENT

Values-based management is an approach to your health care that will support you in personal agency. What we mean by values is what matters most to you, and only you know what that is. Cancer care is meant to be 'person-centred' and that means centred on you and your priorities. And the job of making it happen is shared between you and your cancer care team. This means sharing decision making about your treatment and care with your health care team to the extent that you prefer and working together to tackle challenges as they arise.

WHAT CAN I DO?

Start by being clear about what matters most to you in your treatment and care. Talk with your health care team about your priorities, how involved you want to be in decisions about your care, and who else you want to be involved, such as your partner or other family members or friends. Question lists prepared in advance can help you guide the conversation with your doctor, nurse, or other health professional towards what matters most to you and are a great memory guide. Plan what questions you need answered in advance of your consultation with your doctor or nurse, perhaps with the support of a partner or a close friend. Keeping these questions and answers as notes in a book can help you keep track of conversations and decisions over time. Being informed will help you be more action oriented in how you work with your health care team. Connecting your family doctor to these conversations will help them be ready to support you at home.

TEAMWORK

Cancer care services have become increasingly specialised, as has cancer treatment, and so you likely will find there are people involved in your care from disciplines you might not have heard of or encountered before. Contemporary cancer care is interdisciplinary, which means people from different disciplines work together to get you the best possible outcome. This is where teamwork comes in. Specialists across medicine, surgery, radiology, allied health, and nursing all work together for you.

WHAT CAN I DO?

Find out who is in your cancer care team and keep a list in your notebook of who they are, how they support your care, and how you can contact them if you need them. Ask your doctor or nurse who is the lead person coordinating your care and check who is keeping your family doctor in the loop. If you move to a different treatment approach, you might need to ask these questions again.

VIGILANCE

Vigilance means careful attention. Careful attention to your wellbeing is important to guide and tailor your care to your needs now and as they arise. Your health care team will have a clinical surveillance (i.e., careful attention) plan for you based on the nature of your cancer. For some cancers, this may be time limited, and for other cancers, this may be lifelong. Clinical surveillance from your cancer care team will likely focus on the control of the cancer and management of physical treatment side effects. This should also include regularly checking on your emotional wellbeing by screening for high psychological distress and asking about any concerns that are affecting your quality of life.

As the central actor in your health care and the person who knows how you are going best, you will also need to pay careful attention to your wellbeing. When you have concerns, raise them with your cancer care team or the support people around you.

WHAT CAN I DO?

Let your cancer care team know how you are going both physically and emotionally and what your wellbeing priorities are. The team might not always pick up on your concerns, and they can't read your mind. Don't assume the issues you are concerned about are not important or that your doctor or nurse is not interested or too busy to help. If it matters to you, then it matters to your cancer care team.

Ask your doctor for a survivorship or wellbeing care plan that details your treatments and follow-up checks. Survivorship care plans typically include a treatment summary, a plan about surveillance and follow-up tests, and possible treatment side effects that might occur. Lifestyle tips and wellbeing pointers are also often included. Your doctor may have already provided you with a plan, and if not, we have links to examples in the Resources and Connections section at the end of this book. Discuss your survivorship care plan with your doctor or nurse. You might want to involve your partner or family so you are all across the plan.

STRATEGIES THAT WORK

Your time and energy are valuable. So, any strategies to improve your wellness need to be based on good evidence, in other words be evidence-based. Being evidence-based is about directing your time, energy, and resources to wellness strategies that have strong evidence to support their effectiveness.

Good evidence is available for the effectiveness of a range of emotional and mental wellbeing approaches, and this book includes many of these evidence-based strategies. As discussed earlier, there is excellent evidence for the benefits of exercise medicine or, in other words, a tailored exercise programme. Good nutritional habits are also important. Sexual health support tailored to different treatment effects and for people with different sexual orientations and partner relationships is also an area where good evidence exists about what works, and knowledge here continues to grow.

WHAT CAN I DO?

The tip here is to be discerning about the strategies you use to achieve your wellbeing goals. When you consult practitioners, either personally or by sourcing self-help programmes, check the evidence they have to back up their claims of how this might help you. You might want to check how much experience they have in working with people affected by cancer. Let the people who are supporting you know what your main worries or priorities are, your goals for change, and how you prefer to go about making these changes.

You might ask your cancer care team what wellbeing strategies are important for you in your specific situation. If you are unsure about where to turn for help, consider contacting a credible cancer organisation, such as those listed in the Resources and Connections at the end of this book, and ask for advice. The organisations listed provide a range of different services that include face-to-face services, telehealth, web-based programmes, and self-help guides. Reach out until you find a service that suits you.

It can also be helpful to talk to other people who have had a cancer experience to see what they have found helpful and accessible. Peer support, either through your own social networks or through organised community programmes, can provide a unique source of coping information, emotional support, and practical advice based on shared experience. People often report that this type of support helped them feel less alone in their cancer experience.

FINDING MEANING

Meaning and purpose are about our life story or narrative. Some people find that after cancer, they feel a strong drive for change in some areas of life. They might wish to be more involved in their community and help others facing a similar experience. Advocating for the health and support of others can feel like a way to make some meaning out of all that you might have learnt through your cancer journey. Other people feel a desire to pursue new interests, set new lifestyle goals, or simply seek to live in a more authentic way. It is all about our own personal story and where we want to focus.

WHAT CAN I DO?

We discuss the idea of finding meaning in more detail in the next Chapter. If we think of meaning and purpose as having to do with the story of our lives, then we have a choice. We can change that story if we wish to, or alternatively simply reflect and continue in our daily lives, as changed as it may be from the experience of cancer.

JEFF'S REFLECTION

"Invictus"
"I am the master of my fate
I am the captain of my soul."
William Ernest Henley, 1875

The Wellbeing Essentials Framework (the Framework) emerged from an extensive programme of work with men with prostate cancer, their partners, and the health professionals who care for them. First published in British Journal of Urology International as "Survivorship Essentials", the Framework has evolved as it demonstrated acceptability and efficacy for a broader audience encompassing people across all cancer sites and further to those dealing with a chronic disease, such as diabetes or heart disease.

The first version of the Framework identified a series of six domains, namely, Health Promotion and Agency, Evidence based interventions, Personal Agency, Vigilance, Care Coordination, and Shared Management. Each domain is critical to improving wellbeing after a diagnosis of and treatment for cancer. Importantly, one of those domains, Personal Agency, sits at the centre and is primary to achieving optimal outcomes.

Hence the Henly quote from "Invictus". I quoted the last two lines of the popular poem, where the overarching theme is one of triumph over adversity, resilience, and inner strength. Compelling sentiment when tackling the menace of a cancer diagnosis, and a sentiment consistent with the central tenet of the Framework. Put simply, in the end, you, the patient, are at the centre, and may influence, via whatever means, what sits most comfortably with your demeanour, the trajectories, and the outcome of care.

I Googled survivorship and coping with cancer, and not surprisingly, there are multitudes of stuff out there. One heading, "5 Things they do not tell you about life after cancer", caught my eye. These are:

- Fatigue can last years after treatment. Tick.
- Your sleep habits may change. Tick.
- Anxiety and depression are common. Tick.
- You may struggle with body changes. Tick.
- Treatment may cause late and long-term effects. Tick.

The ticks are mine, not because I was not told about them but because I have experienced them personally. Happily for me no depression, but anxiety for sure. Loss of control and uncertainty about the future and waiting for recurrence will do that to you. Mind you this list of five could be extended extensively, but I will leave that for you to do yourself. What was interesting I thought was a final statement, and I quote, "Survivorship programs offer support even after treatment ends". So, there is recognition that a structured approach to survivorship makes a difference and a concession that the end of treatment is not the end of the challenge. Hence, the focus in the Framework on vigilance and advocacy.

Since being diagnosed every health professional I have come across has genuinely to my mind wanted to help. Just that some do it better than others. Individual differences, circumstances, a bad day after a big night, all these things can influence the experience, but again, I found that putting myself in the equation, being involved with the decision making, the coordination, and working with the professionals improves the process and likelihood of favourable outcomes. Who can help, where can I find them, and how do I get them involved? These are questions I often asked myself and others. And then, I got to work.

Thinking about it, I have sought to balance peaceful acceptance of what is with more proactive, vigorous approaches to influence and advocate, shedding energy along the way. Not always in a planned, rational way, often by dint of circumstance and opportunity and how well I am feeling on any given day. But always in the same prime direction, mastery over my fate. Being aware of the elements and rising to the challenge when it mattered has made all difference for me and those around me.

Let me take you from Henly to Hemingway.

"The world breaks everyone, and then afterward, some are strong in the broken places".

Ernest Hemingway

Here in my afterward, am I stronger in the broken places? I think so, for some; I hope so. Others would be more reliable informants but on the mend. I wish that for you, too – being stronger in the broken places. No matter what the world throws your way.

SUZANNE'S REFLECTION

When Jeff was having intensive treatment, we were given a lot of information, but not a survivorship or wellness plan. I had a red book I kept notes in about the plan, our questions, and the doctors' answers, but to be honest, it was a bit of a muddle. We got there in the end, but I do think if we had drawn up a Wellbeing Essentials Plan, it would have helped.

I think we are now in the Vigilance stage of things. Jeff still has monthly treatment, so he sees his haematologist then, and we do talk about clinical surveillance quite a bit and what this means for us. Surveillance for Jeff is mostly about monthly blood tests to check on his immunity and treatment effects and then responding to these issues as they arise. Learning to live with ongoing surveillance and the uncertainty that sits with that is sometimes a challenge. For me, it comes down to bringing us back to the present moment, how things are right now, and what we can do to live closely to our valued priorities in the present moment.

I guess this connects to the Finding Meaning aspect of wellbeing, and we are certainly setting new lifestyle goals with regard to exercise and nutrition, and frankly, as you age, you need to do this anyway. We are chasing down some long-held hiking goals and making concrete plans to stop talking about it and just do it. Taking control of the narrative.

And we have finished this book. For you.

REFERENCE

1.   Dunn J, Green A, Ralph N, Newton RU, Kneebone A, Frydenberg M, et al. Prostate cancer survivorship essentials framework: Guidelines for practitioners. BJU International. 2021;128(Suppl 3):18–29.

10

IS IT POSSIBLE TO FLOURISH AFTER CANCER?

WHAT DOES IT ALL MEAN? WHY DID THIS HAPPEN TO ME?

The 'why me' and wondering how it is that you or your partner came to be facing cancer is a pretty common response to being in this situation. Cancer is not fair; it strikes people from all walks of life and backgrounds, and living a healthy, pure, and honest life does not make you bulletproof. A threat to life can lead you to wonder about the meaning of life and if 'this is it'. People sometimes ask themselves: 'What sort of person do I want to be? What sort of relationships do I want with others, and what do I want my life to be about?'

There are many philosophical traditions, Western and Eastern, that deal with this question: 'What is the meaning of life, and what is the meaning of my life?' Some people find their religious or spiritual faith helpful, and others find reflection, self-questioning, and the seeking of knowledge an approach that leads to acceptance and strength. This is a personal and very individual path to walk, and there is no one right way to consider what having had cancer or loving someone who has had cancer means to you. It is your journey.

It is important to note that some people do not see their diagnosis as a life changing experience. For them, cancer is just another hurdle

DOI: 10.4324/9781032638843-10

in life to manage and overcome as soon as they can and with the resources they have available. For others, the cancer experience leads them to re-evaluate how they view themselves and the world around them. These are the people who often report positive life changes after struggling with their cancer and treatment. For example, they may feel their relationships with others have deepened or that they are more focused on spending time on their most valued priorities and saying 'no' more often to things that are less important to them.

SHIFTING GOAL POSTS

If the goal posts shifted for you after you found out about the diagnosis of cancer, you may have found that some aspects of your life have changed in a positive way. This is often called 'benefit-finding', which is pretty self-explanatory, or 'post-traumatic growth', which is a little more obscure. Both of these terms refer to when a traumatic event, such as a cancer diagnosis, shakes a person's world up to the point that they find themselves re-evaluating their life direction, personal priorities, relationships, and future goals. This is an introspective and reflective process that can lead to a sense of personal growth and, for some people, decisions to change aspects of their lives. Post-traumatic growth is not confined to the experience of cancer, it can include the experience of war, loss of a loved one, road trauma, or accidents. Any trauma where a person has experienced high levels of emotional distress and a threat to either their own wellbeing or a threat to the wellbeing of people close to them can lead to personal growth. Post-traumatic growth is its own universe in the sense that this positive aspect of change appears to be a separate outcome from the negative. The positive and negative don't cancel each other out, they co-exist.

A common way post-traumatic growth is expressed by people affected by cancer is that they now pay more care and attention to their loved ones and important personal relationships. Alternatively, sometimes a person might find their cancer is the tipping point that leads them to break off a relationship that perhaps has not been right for them for some time. Other people find they develop a new and deeper level of compassion for others and might take up volunteer work for a good cause or try to help others whenever they can. This compassion includes where a person finds within them forgiveness and kindness towards themselves, as well as towards others.

Finding the courage or daring to try new challenges is another way people experience post-traumatic growth. Think of the people you know who have had cancer who take up marathon runs, walks, or cycle trips to raise funds for cancer research as well as to challenge themselves physically. Dragon boating, mountain climbing, motorcycle riding, the list goes on. Another way that people diagnosed with cancer or their loved ones express post-traumatic growth is by reporting a newfound sense of personal strength. This fits with that old saying 'what doesn't kill you, only makes you stronger'. Often people will comment that it wasn't until they were pushed that they realised how much they could deal with. Coming to understand and feel that you can cope with cancer may help you see new strengths in yourself and your abilities to face other challenges that life throws at you.

People who have been diagnosed with cancer often report that their priorities have now shifted. We can all become bogged down in the routine of life – work, paying the bills, commuting. Sometimes it takes something big to awaken us to all the possibilities that life has to offer. After struggling with cancer, some people may decide to spend more time with family and friends and less time at work, and some may decide to pursue life-long dreams that had previously been put on hold. This does not mean that everyone has or even needs to have this type of reaction to their cancer. Just getting through treatment and back to your usual life can be challenging enough.

IS IT POSSIBLE TO FLOURISH AFTER A CANCER DIAGNOSIS?

There are different ways to look at the idea of flourishing (1) and how a person might flourish after cancer. Flourishing is about wellbeing, and within this the idea of finding meaning, deepening personal relationships and thinking about what we value most and pay attention to in our lives, in other words virtue. Human beings are storytellers, and we rewrite our stories across our lives as we see them through happy moments and times of adversity. The story of our lives is in many ways our character, the way we see ourselves, and how we make sense of our lives. And we build and mould this over our lifetime. In a way, adversity can provide a unique opportunity to take stock and think about these aspects of wellbeing, that go beyond physical wellbeing, to think about living our most authentic life. We all do this in different ways; it might be about how we are with the people who are close to us, our spiritual or religious engagement, pursuing self-expression in the arts or music, or moving in a direction we have thought about but not felt able to action. A new challenge or a skill we always wanted to learn. Think about your strengths, the things about yourself you are most proud of, and what matters to you most right now. Are you able to move towards those things, build on them, and use them as the platform for what comes next?

Related to this, people who have been diagnosed with cancer often report that their priorities have now shifted. We can all become bogged down in the routine of life – work, paying the bills, commuting, and keeping up with chores. Sometimes, it takes something big to awaken us to all the possibilities that life has to offer. After struggling with cancer, some people decide to spend more time with family and friends and less time at work, and others may decide to pursue life-long dreams that had previously been put on hold. This does not mean that everyone has or even needs to have this type of reaction to their cancer. Just getting through treatment and back to your usual life can be challenging enough.

After cancer, some people are surprised to find themselves becoming a role model in their circle of friends and their community, and becoming an advocate for better health and wellbeing. Some take up raising awareness and funds for cancer research and offering support to others. Being diagnosed with cancer can open up a new network of friends, activities, and events as a cancer survivor. Joining community groups and even taking part in research are just some of the ways that people may feel they can contribute and give back, as well as gain a sense of belonging with others who understand what they have been through.

Some people proudly, and often, will say, 'I am a cancer survivor', and for them, this means being strong, resilient, and fearless. Others feel that they do not want to define themselves by their cancer and see it more as an experience they have moved past. Again, neither way is right or wrong. What is important is to feel strong and confident about yourself and who you are now. And to write your own story.

A NOTE ABOUT HOPE

It might feel hard at times to feel hopeful. A philosophical view is that hope is believing in the possibility of something good in the future. Others suggest that hope is more than this – it is finding a reason for action to try and find the future good. That it is possible to be realistic about the current situation and the uncertainties and challenges but still find hope. (2) It is all about being open to possibilities.

JEFF'S REFLECTION

"It never hurts to keep looking for sunshine."
Winnie-the-Pooh

Is it possible to flourish after cancer? Why not? Reckon so. Of course! But as for most things, we need to want it and work at it. To me, it seems a naive question because flourishing is what it's all about, isn't it? We all want to flourish. This depends, I suppose, on what you mean by flourishing and what you must do to get there.

We owe much to the ancient Greeks for our modern conception of flourishing. The 5th Edition of the Macquarie English Dictionary speaks to its Greek derivation and then offers 19 alternative definitions, the first focused on being "in a vigorous, prosperous, successful state". In Aristotle's Nicomachean Ethics, considered a classic on the matter of human happiness, he argues that flourishing is the "activity of the soul in accordance with virtue". So, it's not all about strength and success; maybe it's more subtle. Aristotle himself pondered what sort of activities allow a person to live well and even offered some options, for example: a life of pleasure, a life of political activity, or a philosophical life. So, flourishing can mean different things to different people, and there are different pathways to achieve, in Aristotle's words, "the True the Good and the Beautiful", his description of human flourishing. Google it; there are plenty of references and, if you like this sort of thing, a good read. I liked it and found guidance in it, for what that is worth.

In my experience, wellbeing, flourishing if you like, is fluid in time and substance. Depends upon where you are at any given point in time, in life, in treatment, in relationships, in work, etc., etc., and in that context, what exactly is the true, the good, and the beautiful, and where to find it? Tough question. This is where I turn to another well-respected philosopher, Winnie-the-Pooh; we just must keep looking. Brighter days, sunshine days, for all of us, are there for the finding; we just must keep looking.

There is no prescription for flourishing, despite what you might read on the internet. For what it's worth, I found that acceptance was helpful, embracing my new circumstance. So was a belief in myself and those around me, sufficiently so "to give it a go". And purpose, a sense of purpose. Back to work, back to volunteering, checking in with friends, and doing my best to be my best. Virtuous in the Greek sense, living my best life, realising my potential, changed as it was, through altruistic practice and cultivating a 'life of the mind'. I did think about it this way, still do. I find it helpful. Maybe a different approach is needed for you? I don't know.

Something I do know is that wellbeing, happiness, and flourishing, whatever you choose to call it, will not magically appear. Think active pursuit, name it and chase it. Seek it out. The sunshine comes in many forms, sometimes unexpected and in surprising places if you keep looking for it. Sunshine at a price, but a price well within each of us. Seneca, a Stoic, observed: "No person is ever wise by chance". Methinks we might usefully apply this notion to flourishing. Unlikely to happen by chance, you are the master of your destiny in this regard (borrowing from Henly; "Invictus". Again).

Speaking of wisdom, let's round out with more Winnie-the-pooh reasoning:
"I always get to where I am going by walking away from where I have been
Oh, bother! Take that first step!"

SUZANNE'S REFLECTION

I can't say that I have shifted direction as a result of Jeff's cancer. I did set some new goals. The experience was quite shattering, and I wanted to pay service to it in some way. Agreeing to do this book was part of that for me and for us. Honouring our experience. It has led me to think more about my values and what I contribute to others around me, as a parent and grandparent and as a colleague and friend. We all get a bit wrapped up in our own internal worlds, and I am trying to do that less.

As a therapist working with people with cancer, I think it has deepened my understanding of that experience, and I hope it has made me more helpful to the people I see. I think it makes me notice more about my patients' experiences and be more flexible in my approach. And I learn from my patients. They are a gift.

There is a quote Jeff shared with me recently from Henry David Thoreau: "The question is not what you look at, but what you see." I am hoping that when I am with my patients, I truly see them, their pain, and their beauty and do my best to walk with them on their path.

For my lovely husband, I see his courage every day; no matter how sick he is, fatigued, in pain, or unwell, he gets up, does the needful, and keeps going. He finds hope, and in seeing him, I do as well, alongside the tears.

REFERENCES

1. Logan AC, Berman BM, Prescott SL. Vitality revisited: The evolving concept of flourishing and its relevance to personal and public health. International Journal of Environmental Research and Public Health. 2023;20(6).
2. Case B, Vanderweele T. The power of hope amid an epidemic of despair. Overland Park, KS: Made to Flourish; 2024. Available from: https://commongoodmag.com/the-power-of-hope-amid-an-epidemic-of-despair/.

RESOURCES AND CONNECTIONS

Many countries have community-based cancer organisations that provide information and support for people living with cancer and their families. Some of these cover all cancer types, and some are tailored to specific cancer types. What follows is a brief list of some organisations in different countries that offer cancer support or information. This is not an exhaustive list, and we advise you to talk to your health care team for guidance about the services most suitable for you. For medical or treatment questions, your doctor is the best first point of call for advice that is personalised to your situation. Contact details were accurate at the time of printing.

SOURCES OF INFORMATION AND SUPPORT

United Kingdom

https://www.cancerresearchuk.org Cancer Research UK provides detailed information about different cancers and their treatment backed up by a nurse freephone helpline. They also offer a fully moderated forum called Cancer Chat, where you can talk to others affected by cancer, share experiences, and get support.

https://www.maggies.org/cancer-support Maggie's provides information and support for people with cancer and their carers. This includes courses and workshops designed to help you learn about living well with cancer, support groups, and Benefits Advisors to provide guidance on entitlements and practical help.

https://www.macmillan.org.uk/ Macmillan Cancer Support provides support for people with cancer and their carers through a Support Line (seven days, 8 am–8 pm), email, and online chat with trained cancer information advisors. An online community, free specialist counselling, peer support buddies, and online information can provide reassurance and direction to further resources on a range of topics.

https://cancersupportuk.org/ Cancer Support UK provides information, education, and support about coping with a cancer diagnosis. The six-week Cancer Coach eLearning programme provides education about common emotional challenges post-treatment. A one-off Cancer Coach Focus Forwards workshop gives a chance to learn and chat with others who have just completed treatment, while long-term peer support in facilitated groups is also available.

https://www.mariecurie.org.uk/ Marie Curie provides clinical and emotional care during palliative and end-of-life stages. As well as a phone helpline, Marie Curie can support palliative care in a hospice or at home, and companion volunteers provide emotional and practical companionship approaching the end of life. Comprehensive information is available online.

https://www.nhs.uk/conditions/cancer/ The NHS provide information on a range of specific cancers, a search platform for local cancer support services, and links to cancer-specific charities and information.

https://prostatecanceruk.org/ Prostate Cancer UK provides specific advice and support for men with prostate cancer and their families. A specialist prostate cancer nurse phoneline is available, as well as opportunities to contact via email, online chat, or talk to peers in an online community. Information about prostate cancer risk, signs, and symptoms for newly diagnosed men and those living with prostate cancer is available.

https://www.prostatescotland.org.uk/ Prostate Scotland provides education about prostate cancer risk and disease and support to navigate prostate cancer for those who have been diagnosed. The COMPASS programme provides a range of support services, including a Living Well with Prostate Cancer Course, a Prostate Scotland Cancer Navigator App, Cancer Support Specialists, and a free exercise programme.

https://roycastle.org/about-us/ The Roy Castle Lung Foundation assists those with lung cancer from diagnosis to survivorship and end-of-life care. In addition to comprehensive information about lung cancer, from risk factors through to diagnosis, treatment, and palliation, the Foundation offers a range of services, including nurse consultations, 'Keep in Touch' support service, group and online support, smoking cessation support, a will-writing service, and patient grants for treatment-related costs.

https://breastcancernow.org/ Breast Cancer Now is a charity that engages in research and support services to support patients navigating breast cancer care for primary and secondary breast cancers. Online Speakers Live sessions provide education about primary breast cancer topics. Opportunities to engage with others also experiencing breast cancer include 'Someone Like Me', a one-to-one email or phone support service connecting current patients with volunteers that have finished their treatment to provide support and advice. The 'Younger Women Together' online and in-person sessions also deliver education and peer support opportunities tailored to younger women with breast cancer aged 20 to 45 years.

Australia

https://www.cancer.org.au/ The *Cancer Council Helpline* is a free, confidential telephone information and support service run by Cancer Councils in each state and territory in Australia. Specially trained staff are available to answer questions about cancer and provide support.

Call 13 11 20 (local call cost from anywhere in Australia, but mobile calls are charged at mobile rates), open between 9 am and 5 pm, Monday to Friday; however, some states have extended hours. The Cancer Council also provides cancer information for specific communities, such as First Nations people and Culturally and Linguistically Diverse people, and a search platform for local services.

https://www.pcfa.org.au/ The Prostate Cancer Foundation of Australia is Australia's leading community-based organisation for prostate cancer research, awareness, and support. The PCFA website includes general and detailed information about prostate cancer risk, screening, and treatment, which is guided by the Prostate Cancer Survivorship Essentials Framework. Comprehensive support options are available, including funded Prostate Cancer Specialist Nurses and selected locations, Prostate Cancer Specialist Telenursing Service, Counselling Service, support groups, and the MatesCONNECT programme for phone-based peer support. A Prostate Cancer Survivorship Toolkit guides patients on how to access information and support services to live well with prostate cancer.

https://lungfoundation.com.au/ Lung Foundation Australia focuses on information and support for those with lung disease, including cancer. Information and support services are available, including support groups, exercise programmes, webinars, and advice for living with a chronic lung disease. Lung Cancer Support nurses provide cancer-specific support, while the Lung Cancer Search and Rescue campaign aims to provide reliable information about living with lung cancer from survivors.

https://www.bcna.org.au/ The Breast Cancer Network Australia brings together English and multi-lingual resources in audio and text forms for women experiencing breast cancer in their Information & Resource Hub. Specific information is available for breast cancer and men, young people, LGBTQI+ people, First Nations peoples, and rural patients. A Helpline is available for advice and support, as well as the 'My Care Kit' for those who have undergone breast cancer surgery and 'My Decision' resource to support information decision making about treatment, breast reconstruction, and fertility.

https://www.ovariancancer.net.au/ Ovarian Cancer Australia supports people with ovarian cancer by delivering care, support, and advocacy for women with ovarian cancer. In addition to information on all aspects of ovarian cancer, the online CareHub directs patients to additional resources, while the Teal Support Program aims to improve care continuity and meet the individual needs of patients, family, and friends.

New Zealand

https://www.cancer.org.nz/ The *Cancer Society of New Zealand* has a free Cancer Information Helpline, 0800 CANCER (226 237), which supplies booklets, information sheets, and other information resources which can also be downloaded directly from their website.

North America

https://www.cancer.org/ The American Cancer Society provides a cancer helpline service, cancer navigation service, support groups, and practical services such as accommodation and transport for treatment. Information about selected specific cancers and phases of cancer management from diagnosis to palliative care are also available.

https://www.pcf.org/ The Prostate Cancer Foundation aims to ensure that men are managed by the right team, are diagnosed with the right tests, and are provided the right treatment specific to their needs and situation. Patient navigation services help to connect patients with local providers, improve opportunities for peer support through support groups, and education through online resources and webinars. Specific information about topics of interest for prostate cancer patients is also available.

https://www.komen.org/ Komen supports women with breast cancer in the United States and their families, in addition to research and policy advocacy work. Komen operates a telephone helpline, a Patient Care Centre, advice on participating in clinical trials, and practical assistance and advice regarding the financial impacts of living with breast cancer.

Canada

https://cancer.ca/en/ The Canadian Cancer Society provides information about a broad range of cancer types, as well as treatment types and clinical trials. A toll-free phone line and live chat are available for immediate assistance.

CANCER SURVIVORSHIP CARE PLANS

https://prostate.org.au/my-cancer-wellbeing-plan This care plan has been developed as a general cancer survivorship plan that can be adapted to fit a person's needs. It is closely aligned to the Wellbeing Essentials framework and is designed to be completed together with your cancer care team. The plan can be used to record your cancer treatment plan, to identify your key concerns, and set wellbeing priorities and actions to work towards these.

https://www.mycareplan.org.au/ This care plan discusses health risks people may face as a result of cancer and its treatment. Individual risks depend on the type of treatment a person has received.

https://www.cancer.org/cancer/survivorship/long-term-health-concerns/survivorship-care-plans.html/ The ASCO Survivorship Care Plan includes details about what someone might need for follow-up after treatment. This includes check-ups, surveillance, and the possible long-term side effects of treatment. It also includes options for healthy living.

https://www.pancare.eu/pancarefollowup-care-intervention-replication-manual/survivorship-care-plan-template/ The PanCare FollowUp Survivorship Care Plan provides patients with a summary of their diagnosis and treatments, standard recommendations for long-term follow-up care, and individualised recommendations for long-term follow-up care.

https://oncolife.oncolink.org/ The OncoLife online tool, maintained by PennMedicine, helps cancer survivors to develop their own survivorship care plan using a short questionnaire that can then be reviewed with their clinicians. The tool offers both patient and healthcare provider versions of the questionnaire and care plan.

https://www.sahealth.sa.gov.au/ | Survivorship Framework Implementation Resources This plan records information about your cancer, treatment, and supportive services you have accessed. It helps you and your healthcare provider to understand your current issues or future priorities, what is most important to you, and a plan for how to achieve your goals. It is designed to be shared with members of your broader healthcare team, including your GP, to facilitate handover of care from your specialist provider.

https://www.esmo.org/content/download/117593/2061518/ 1/ESMO-Patient-Guide-Survivorship.pdf The European Society for Medical Oncology provides a detailed patient guide to survivorship, including extensive information on all aspects of survivorship and informed by the ESMO Clinical Practice Guidelines. The guide also includes a survivorship checklist, care plan, and treatment summary for patients and clinicians.

CANCER-SPECIFIC SURVIVORSHIP CARE PLANS ARE ALSO AVAILABLE, SUCH AS:

Prostate cancer

https://www.pcfa.org.au/media/umbbmgwi/my-wellbeing-plan-2024.pdf

Gastro-intestinal cancer

https://www.gicancersalliance.org/wp-content/uploads/2017/11/ GICA_SurvivorshipCarePlan_web-form.pdf/

Early breast cancer

https://www.canceraustralia.gov.au/sites/default/files/publications/shared-care-plan/pdf/scbfs_ebc_shared_care_plan_int.pdf

Hodgkin's Lymphoma

https://www.hodgkinsinternational.com/wp-content/uploads/2023/03/hi_survivorship_plan_rev._6-3-c.pdf

Leukaemia and lymphoma (Adult, Young Adult, and Children and Adolescent versions)

https://www.lls.org/managing-your-cancer/survivorship-workbook

Lung cancer

https://society.asco.org/sites/new-www.asco.org/files/content-files/practice-patients/documents/2024-nsclc-treatment-summary-and-survivorship-care-plan.docx

OTHER BOOKS BY THESE AUTHORS

Chambers S. Facing the tiger: A survivorship guide for men with prostate cancer and their partners. Australian Academic Press; 2020. ISBN 978-1925644425.

Chambers S, Dunn J. The health professionals guide to delivering psychological care for adults with cancer. Australian Academic Press; 2023. ISBN 9781925644654.

Chambers S, Heneka N, Dunn J. The health professionals guide to delivering psychological care for men with prostate cancer. Australian Academic Press; 2021. ISBN 9781925644555.

For Product Safety Concerns and Information please contact our EU
representative GPSR@taylorandfrancis.com
Taylor & Francis Verlag GmbH, Kaufingerstraße 24, 80331 München, Germany